LACTATION FOR
THE REST OF US

T0304483

of related interest

Supporting Queer Birth
A Book for Birth Professionals and Parents
AJ Silver
ISBN 978 1 83997 045 0
eISBN 978 1 83997 046 7

The Trans Guide to Mental Health and Well-Being
Katy Lees
ISBN 978 1 78775 526 0
eISBN 978 1 78775 527 7

Gender Confirmation Surgery
A Guide for Trans and Non-Binary People
Edward Whelan
ISBN 978 1 83997 096 2
eISBN 978 1 83997 097 9

Lactation for the Rest of Us

A Guide for Queer and Trans Parents and Helpers

Jacob Engelsman, IBCLC

Foreword by Dr. Izzy Lowell

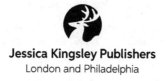

Jessica Kingsley Publishers
London and Philadelphia

First published in Great Britain in 2025 by Jessica Kingsley Publishers
An imprint of John Murray Press

1

Copyright © Jacob Engelsman 2025
Foreword copyright © Dr. Izzy Lowell 2025

The information contained in this book is not intended to replace the services
of trained medical professionals or to be a substitute for medical advice. You
are advised to consult a doctor on any matters relating to your health, and in
particular on any matters that may require diagnosis or medical attention.

A CIP catalogue record for this title is available from the British Library and
the Library of Congress

ISBN 978 1 80501 191 0
eISBN 978 1 80501 192 7

Printed and bound in the United States by Integrated Books International

Jessica Kingsley Publishers' policy is to use papers that are natural, renewable
and recyclable products and made from wood grown in sustainable forests.
The logging and manufacturing processes are expected to conform to the
environmental regulations of the country of origin.

Jessica Kingsley Publishers
Carmelite House
50 Victoria Embankment
London EC4Y 0DZ

www.jkp.com

John Murray Press
Part of Hodder & Stoughton Limited
An Hachette UK Company

The authorised representative in the EEA is Hachette Ireland,
8 Castlecourt Centre, Dublin 15, D15 XTP3, Ireland (email: info@hbgi.ie)

This book is dedicated to my spouse, who is the tree for my ivy.

Contents

PART 2: HOW TO MAKE MILK WITHOUT BEING PREGNANT

PART 3: GENERAL LACTATION INFORMATION

Foreword

Finally, it is here: a book about lactation written for everyone—including all of us who do not identify as women or mothers—and partners of all genders.

So many trans and nonbinary people struggle to find affirming medical care and advice about the most basic things. It is especially hard to find support and guidance about lactation if you do not fit into the typical body or role of "mother." This comprehensive guide covers the physiology of how all bodies can make milk, techniques and medications to assist with lactation, and trans and nonbinary focused answers to questions cisgender people never even considered.

Lactation can be an amazing, life-changing experience that connects us with our children like nothing else. It can also be challenging, frustrating, exhausting, and unfortunately highly gendered by society. In this book, we are all affirmed and supported. We get to hear about the experiences of others who have gone through it, the challenges, failures, successes, and wisdom they have to offer. You are not alone in this book.

I am the founder of QueerMed, a telemedicine practice providing hormone therapy for transgender and nonbinary people of all ages across the country. I often get questions from patients I can't answer, and I have to reply, "We just don't have much data on this; no one has studied that in trans/nonbinary people." Now we have a comprehensive, evidence-based book by an International Board Certified Lactation Consultant for all genders, focused on those of us who have been excluded from typical medical literature. All of the rest of us who may not identify as cisgender will be affirmed and informed. Whether you are giving birth to a baby, want to lactate, or are supporting a partner in these endeavors, this book will guide you on the incredible journey.

Dr. Izzy Lowell (she/her)
JANUARY 15, 2024

Author's note: A few weeks after I received the foreword from Dr. Lowell, a fire that had occurred at the QueerMed office was determined to be an act of arson. As of this writing, an FBI investigation is still ongoing (Whisenhunt & Atlanta First News Staff, 2024).

Introduction

The most important thing you need to know about this book is that it will never assume your sex, gender, sexuality, or relationship to any (current or future) baby.

When referring to the parents and helpers for whom this book was written, I use terms like parent, chestfeeding, bodyfeeding, lactation, gestation, and human milk. These are terms that can apply to anyone, regardless of their current, past, or future gender or sexuality. This approach to lactation care without assuming gender is something I have started referring to as *postgender* lactation support. This is not to say that this book does not contain words like *nursing*, *breastfeeding*, and *mother*. You will find them in interviews and quotations from other people and literature where I feel it's very important that exact wording be used. I hope you will bear with me through these interludes.

I was once asked, if I had a magic wand and could change the world in any way, what would I do? The subject of the interview was gender diversity, otherwise my answer probably would have had something to do with sandwiches (I know who I am), but the answer I came up with was: I would completely get rid of the concept of gender, just erase it from everyone's mind. Not change human physiology or anatomy, just nix the idea that those kinds of traits divide people in any meaningful way. I imagine a world where some people are just thought of as having the necessary organs to gestate babies and some people choose to lactate the same way that some people have excellent vision and some choose to learn yoga, or knit; but having these abilities and skills doesn't imply having other abilities or limitations—that, to me, would be a more ideal world.

What if, instead of treating gender as something like height or weight—something that can often be determined by looking at a person—we treated it as a more variable identifier, like a religion or nationality? Something that maybe you can get a clue of by the way someone dresses or behaves but you would never second guess a person when they tell you you're incorrect.

After thousands of years of written history you might be inclined to think that there are enough books on human lactation. The problem, as I saw it, is that these books were almost all written for the same audience. Which is to say, cis women who just gave birth. Now, with the 21st century well under way and the wonders of global communication at our fingertips, it seems the time has come for a lactation book for, well, the rest of us, whether that is people who have just given birth but are not women, people whose partner has just had a baby, people who have a baby by adoption, surrogacy, or any of the other ways people end up with babies these days.

To ensure that this book does not reflect only one perspective, I've included information and excerpts from interviews with birth and lactation professionals throughout the book. You may notice that there are parts where the contributors seem to disagree with each other about various aspects of queerness or lactation. This just goes to show that there is no single right way to be a queer person or a parent, and there is still so much we are learning about the human body. These are lactation and birth professionals I spoke to:

- AJ Silver (they/them) is a postnatal doula and educator based in the UK. They are the founder of Queer Birth Club, an organization that teaches lesbian, gay, bisexual, transgender, queer, intersex, asexual and others (LGBTQIA+) competency for lactation and birth professionals. They are also the author of *Supporting Queer Birth* and *Supporting Fat Birth*.

- Anissa (they/them) is a midwife at Metroplex Midwifery in Dallas, Texas, who gave birth a few years ago and offered their wonderful insight into lactation as a nonbinary person.

- Bryna Hayden (they/them) and I first met at the US Lactation Consultant Association conference in 2022, where they spoke on the specifics of supporting trans feminine people who induce lactation. We were the only two people speaking on LGBTQIA+-specific issues that year, and I immediately knew that I would need to interview them for this project.

- Kristin-Cole Cavuto (she/he/they) is an International Board Certified Lactation Consultant and former La Leche League leader based in New Jersey. They are one of the many people I spoke to for this book who were inspired by their personal lactation experience to become a lactation professional.

- Rebekah (she/her) has experience personally inducing lactation as well as a career as a lactation consultant where she helps many families with the same.

- Victoria Facelli (she/her) is the author of *Feed the Baby: An Inclusive Guide to Nursing, Bottle-Feeding & Everything in Between* (2023) and was gracious enough to speak with me about her experiences with her daughter and the process of letting go of expectations.

Since all the research in the world cannot replicate the actual experience of actually doing something, I also reached out to several parents who induced lactation, with varying degrees of success. Unsurprisingly, all of the lactation professionals I spoke with also have experience as lactating parents, which was included where appropriate.

This book is divided into collections of essays and collections of pertinent questions. Since this book is for queer parents, I have not included an explanation of why this book is needed. Queer people will already know why and do not need to be reminded. Cis het readers are welcome, but I am writing with the assumption that you are already a person who strives to be an ally.

- Part 1 contains the information that sets this book apart from other lactation guides. Here you will find information particularly relevant to gestational parents in the nonbinary or transmasc communities. The information in these chapters will also be beneficial to all parents, however, with the final chapter specifically for non-lactating parents.

- Part 2 focuses on inducing lactation, which I expect may either be the main reason you are looking at this book, or you may think it is totally irrelevant to your needs. However, there is a lot for all parents to learn in this section about managing goals and expectations. This also includes a thorough discussion of pumps.

- Part 3 opens with a chapter detailing how exactly the human body makes milk during and after pregnancy. This is followed by a series of questions which I have received frequently as a lactation professional and which will be beneficial to all parents or partners, regardless of sex, gender, sexuality, or relationship status. Also included is an excerpt from one of my interviews on handling chestfeeding when you have to stop sooner than planned.

- I have given the closing words to people who have experience as lactating parents and had advice to share, but chose not to be interviewed.

- I have also included two appendices. The first is an essay for anyone interested in lactation in the cis male community, which I felt was important to include to round out "the rest of us." The second is an essay on how and why someone might wish to become a lactation consultant. In my experience, when learning about lactation for the first time is when most become interested in joining our ranks.

Lactation consultants love to talk about how we are the only health-care providers who, at each consultation, have two patients: the child and the parent. While we all get into this field because we want to help people in general, in my experience the main focus of many lactation practices is women helping women. Which is, of course, both an incredibly worthy endeavor and statistically correct. The groups of people who become lactation consultants and people who give birth are both almost exclusively women. Almost. If I'm being honest though, in my heart, I take care of babies. Part of it may be that because I don't have children of my own, all I want to do is help people with theirs. A bigger part of it, however, is that I honestly believe that infants are the best any of us can ever hope to be. I'll close with this quote from the artist Keith Haring: "Babies represent the possibility of the future, the understanding of perfection, how perfect we could be. There is nothing negative about a baby, ever" (Thompson, 1990).

PART 1

QUEER AND TRANS MASC LACTATION CONCERNS

CHAPTER 1

Introduction to Lactation

Much of the information and advertisements new parents receive seems to enforce a false dichotomy—babies who *exclusively* receive their parent's milk and babies who *never* receive their parent's milk. There is messaging that implicitly (and sometimes explicitly) states that your baby is doomed to a life of "artificial feeding" if you are unable to produce enough milk to meet *all* of your baby's caloric needs. I'd like to bring more nuance to this conversation and help you understand your options along your feeding journey, such that you can make choices that serve both you and your baby.

This messaging acts as if lactation exists in a vacuum where everything is always the same, which is, on its face, absurd. Even in the best circumstances, all sorts of difficulties can arise. AJ graciously provides us with an example from their own life where you can see the problem is one that likely affects many people:

> They lost 14% of their birth weight at day 10. We were taken back to hospital—content warning for poorly babies here—because they were poorly. You know, they weren't getting enough and I didn't know what the fuck I was doing. My mom is one of nine, you know, I'm one of 30 cousins or whatever. There was never any shortage of babies and wee-uns running around when I was a kid but in terms of feeding a baby? No, I'd never seen anybody do that.

You read *What to Expect…* and all those kinds of cliché books but when you're a 23-year-old first-time parent? When the healthcare assistant passed me the baby, I was like, I didn't even know which way her feet had to go.

And then there are the specific difficulties faced by queer and trans populations, such as gender dysphoria, the technical aspects of having multiple lactating parents, and other people's reactions. These may be reactions from various phobic populations or from members of your own community who may accuse you of straight-assimilation, especially if you and your partner had the necessary body parts to conceive a child without intervention. If you find yourself worried about being "queer enough," remember these words from Kristin-Cole:

If somebody is queer, they're queer, no matter who they're in a relationship with. Bi and pansexuality exist and are very, very, very queer; being nonbinary is very, very, very queer. Not all trans people go on T and grow beards, and not all people who are super, super, super queer have partners that have the same junk as them.

And when we see those people as clients, we need to recognize their queerness. It's so important. It's so important. I see lots and lots and lots of, you know, "opposite sex queer couples," and it's so important that I'm with them in their queerness, that they're not there as a straight couple. Because they've been treated like that, and it's so disheartening and so soul crushing, especially in hospitals, giving birth, and obstetricians offices, midwives offices. Being constantly looked at as a straight couple when you're not is awful. It's not a good feeling.

When we look at health disparities, bisexuals are right up there with trans people in terms of health disparities based on just how they're treated, so it's real. Biphobia and panphobia are physically killing people. So yeah, I always want to bring that up to remind everyone that just because, you know, just because you have two people who were born with different junk doesn't necessarily mean they're heterosexual or cis for that matter.

I don't want to overload you with too much data on the subject, but I will include one piece of evidence on mental health in the bisexual community to demonstrate the point:

...lifetime rates of mood/anxiety disorders were higher among bisexual-identified women (58.7% for mood disorders, 57.8% for anxiety disorders) compared to lesbians (44.4% for mood disorders, 40.8% for anxiety disorders) and heterosexual women (30.5% for mood disorders, 31.3% for anxiety disorders). Lifetime rates of mood/anxiety disorders were also higher among bisexual-identified men (36.9% for mood disorders, 38.7% for anxiety disorders) compared to heterosexual men (19.8% for mood disorders, 18.6% for anxiety disorders), but rates were similar to gay men (42.3% for mood disorders, 41.2% for anxiety disorders). (Feinstein & Dyar, 2017)

If you're pregnant as you are reading this book, you might be thinking any number of things from, "I'm barely getting through this pregnancy, there's no way I'm going to be able to latch the baby" to, "I definitely want my baby to only have my milk for as long as possible." These may end up shifting and changing as time goes on, and I invite you to stay open as you learn more about lactation, your preferences and insights, and especially as you adjust to life with your baby. That is both common and normal.

The mental health of new parents is a very important consideration as they plan for and experience feeding, and it is often overlooked. If producing milk causes emotional, psychological, or physiological distress, then ceasing production is a perfectly reasonable option which may be worth considering. To paraphrase something a mentor often said to me, no amount of milk makes up for having a clinically depressed parent. As much as I want you to have access to accurate information about lactation, I want you to feel empowered to make the choices that help you feel as healthy as possible.

After about 40 weeks of pregnancy, most people have an idea about whether they definitely do or definitely do not want to lactate. If you are a person who believes lactation will be right for you or you are trying to stay open and curious about chestfeeding, I hope this book will provide you with a foundation of knowledge to begin your journey and navigate challenges as they arise.

While it is almost universally considered true that your milk is the ideal food for your baby, an all-or-nothing perspective is unhelpful and untrue. There are many ways and combinations to feed your baby, and all of them are valid. Human milk, no matter how much or how little you produce, is great for your child but the expression, "letting perfect be the enemy of good" comes to mind. There is no such thing as a "perfect" feeding journey, just the choices that are best for you and your family.

In fact, it could be surmised that if *any* amount of formula is detrimental to your baby (I'm not saying that's true, just that it is a thing people say), then it could also be said that *any* amount of human milk is good for your baby. Maybe you will be producing half the milk your baby needs, or you have one or more partners who want to help with feeding, or lactation is wreaking havoc on your emotional state and you decide to integrate formula or donor milk. In any of these scenarios and many others, you are learning how you want to feed your baby, and that's great. Good job!

I encourage you to trust yourself and what you know to be right and true for your body and mind as you navigate your unique feeding journey. I also encourage families to acknowledge that bodyfeeding is a nonlinear process and requires practice. It is time consuming, physically demanding, and means more changes to your physical body. Feeding can also be a connecting, empowering, and fascinating experience for some parents. Remember that you are not alone in whatever choices you are making; there are professionals and fellow parents who can offer support along the way.

CHAPTER 2

FAQs from Nonbinary and Trans Masc Patients

As an IBCLC focused on the needs of queer and trans parents, I know that there are many questions and discussion points that come up repeatedly when I'm talking with either queer/trans parents (or parents to be) or other professionals interested in learning about my specific fields. In this chapter, I address the most frequently asked questions as well as some which are less frequent but equally important. Some of these questions will apply to all gestational parents and some will only apply to a few of you. Still, I encourage everyone to read through all of them, as you might learn something you didn't know you were missing. Lactation can be an intricate journey, and the more knowledge you have the better!

You mention being an IBCLC. What is that? Are you a doctor or nurse?

IBCLC stands for International Board Certified Lactation Consultant, which is a certification that requires specific training, clinicals, and a rigorous exam. This is the most extensive set of education requirements in the lactation field. Because there is no standardized licensure for folks who call themselves "lactation consultants," people with a wide range of experiences and training (or none at all) may be using this term, and, legally, it's true. (At the time of writing, three states in the US license lactation consultants.) While there is a lot of continuing education for IBCLCs that focuses on gender diverse families, such education is not mandatory and I encourage you to vet potential lactation consultants as you would other medical professionals. A simple question to ask would be, "Has any of your continuing education focused on care for LGBTQIA+ clients?" If it has, you're probably good to go, and if they mention classes or lectures by me, or any of my contributors (Bryna Hayden, Kristin-Cole Cavuto, and AJ Silver in particular are prolific speakers), you should be in good hands.

A person with the IBCLC certification may also be a doctor, nurse, doula, or other birth or infant care professional, but not necessarily. Many IBCLCs work in private practice or specialized lactation clinics. Large hospitals tend to have IBCLCs on staff, and occasionally, a pediatrician or obstetrician may have an IBCLC on staff. In these cases, they tend to be registered nurses who have the additional certification.

Is there anything I can do ahead of time to help chestfeeding go more smoothly?

When folks ask about this I often invite them to think about managing expectations for how chestfeeding will go. What does "go more smoothly" mean to you? If you expect it to be very easy and that everything will just come naturally, you could be setting yourself up for frustration after the baby arrives. On the other hand, if you expect it to be painful, difficult, and unenjoyable for you and the baby, you may create a self-fulfilling prophecy. *Cortisol* (a stress hormone) can cause a delay or decrease in milk production, so focusing on being flexible and open to learning can be beneficial in multiple ways.

If the very idea or act of latching your child is causing you to panic or creates unmanageable dysphoria, accepting that fact can be the most compassionate decision you make for yourself and your family. In this case, create an alternate feeding plan (potentially with a lactation consultant) and talk with a therapist or trusted friend ahead of time to try and work through your concerns. The alternate feeding plan could involve donor milk or formula, or perhaps a partner is interested in inducing lactation?

Now, with these considerations in mind, here are some concrete steps you can take to proactively prepare for your feeding journey:

- *Learn and educate yourself.* You're here, so good job, you! Unfortunately, most of the books and workshops on queer birth and lactation are geared towards professionals, but for more information on pregnancy and birth I would recommend *Queer Conception* by Kristin L. Kali (2022). If you're seeking additional lactation information, I would check out *Feed the Baby*, by Victoria Facelli (2023), who I also interviewed for this book. For personal support, you may be able to find local parenting groups if you are in a large enough area.

- *Create a dedicated feeding area.* If possible, have a specific chair, side of the couch, or area where you're going to do the pumping and feeding as soon as you get home from the hospital or birth center. This is your area now. Make sure it has a little side table, snacks, and water. If you like watching TV, have it by the TV. Maybe you have a dedicated speaker that lives there. Keep your pump in this area, a phone charger, maybe some comfort reading material, nipple ointment and pads, and anything else that may be comforting or distracting for you.

- *Establish a support team.* We all have people who mean well, but it's good to have an idea of the local friends and family who will actually be helpful when the new baby arrives:

people who have newborn experience, and your ride-or-die friends. This includes birth and lactation professionals who are queer themselves, or at least come recommended by the community. You may never need a lactation consultant, but you'll have a much better time if you decide early who they're going to be rather than trying to find a good one while you're in the thick of it.

- *Start prenatal hand expression.* Hand expression is using your hands to massage your chest and express colostrum, which is a special kind of early milk that is thick and kind of gold in color. You'll often see it referred to as *liquid gold.* Colostrum is very beneficial to the newborn's digestive system and provides antibodies for their immune system.

  If you can start expressing a few weeks before your due date, you can collect colostrum in little syringes that you can buy at a pharmacy. Label these with the date and store them in the freezer until you begin laboring. This is a good way to really get in touch with your own body, and it can be a big confidence builder, but keep in mind that it may take a few tries before you get anything.

  The National Health Service in the UK recommends prenatal hand expression particularly for people whose babies may have trouble getting enough food (e.g. multiples, babies with a cleft palate or Down syndrome, or babies who are likely to have a stay in the neonatal intensive care unit) and it's a good way to get the ball rolling for people who may have difficulty producing enough milk (e.g. parents with polycystic ovary syndrome (PCOS), diabetes, or who have had any kind of chest surgery). There's no commitment to using hand expression long term; you can try it out for a little while and if you find it's kind of a bother or more emotionally harmful than helpful, you can just stop.

I talk about the specific technique in Chapter 5 under "Massaging" in Step 2. The difference here is that you will also be manipulating your nipple to specifically try to draw milk out.

You shouldn't begin prenatal hand expression if your midwife or doctor has told you that you are at a particular risk for premature labor (Jones & Warner, 2023).

How long will I need to do this for?

This answer assumes that you want to be lactating at all. Information on how to cease lactation as soon as possible can be found later in this chapter.

Sometimes when people ask this question, they are looking for more of a philosophical or spiritual answer than a straightforward recommendation. If that's you, the answer is that you should do this for as long as *both you and the baby* want to. You have as much right to a vote on this as the baby does, and bodyfeeding has to be unanimous. Your long-term mental health is just as important as the baby's microbiome. And if that choice is making you feel selfish, consider that your continued mental health will help your child well past infancy.

A more linear answer is that although there will never stop being some benefit to the baby getting your milk, everyone weans eventually. Here are some concrete goals you might consider:

- *One week:* If you really want to give chestfeeding a go but are unsure how you'll feel when it's actually happening, make your goal just to give your baby colostrum, the nutrient and antibody-dense precursor to milk.

- *One-to-six months:* For most aspects of childcare, there are as many opinions about the "proper" thing to do as there are people speaking, which is why it's so noteworthy that there is as close to a consensus on this matter as you ever see in the scientific community. The American Academy of Pediatrics (AAP), National Health Service (NHS), and World Health Organization (WHO), among many others, all recommend that babies have nothing but human milk for at least the first six months of life (Meek & Noble, 2022; National Health Service, 2020; World Health Organization, 2021).

- *Two years +:* If those first six months go well for you and you're feeling ambitious, the same organizations recommend feeding a combination of milk and solid foods for at least two years. We've all heard stories of people chestfeeding for years beyond that so I'll go ahead and reiterate my initial answer: do it for as long as both you and the baby want to. Anissa shares their experience of deciding to wean when it became apparent that someone was becoming overly frustrated with the experience:

> We nursed for about two-and-a-half years. That was great. I probably would have even gone longer but the child and I were having a little bit of conflict about it. She was getting really mad that there wasn't as much milk as there used to be. She would yell at me and hit me while we were nursing so eventually I was like, "Okay, I think we need to taper down a little bit." We did and it went okay.

You can stop as early as you need to, but consider that once you stop making milk, relactating is possible but not guaranteed. As we know, other people will have opinions on how long you choose to chestfeed your baby and if you are very unlucky you will hear about those opinions. If this happens to you and you need some reassurance, I've provided some opinions from actual professionals to counterbalance others you may be hearing. Feel free to mark this page. As AJ says:

> I think that there's this assumption in the UK predominantly that breastfeeding is okay, as long as we're talking about just transference of calories. Because there's so much that comes out when babies hit six months, a year, two years. All over the Global North and in the western world entirely we hear, "Oh well, they can have food now and you're doing it for yourself, not the baby." And so it's getting people to understand that it's so much more than that. It's not just the transference of calories. It is so much more and there are so many more goals—outside, "I want to be the sole purpose that my baby lives for six months," which is a fair goal, that's a fine goal. Of course, that's a grand goal. But there's so much more joy in the gray area.

Regarding the mental health aspects, consider that pumping and bottle feeding may be beneficial to the mental and emotional well-being of the baby's other parents, as Victoria explains:

> I had a client who was a trans dad, his wife carried and she had PCOS and low production. So they had a lot of donor milk and for him, bottle feeding that donor milk, which they called *daddy milk*, was great for their family, was really gender affirming for him, and really affirming in parentage.
>
> My family lives more egalitarian and balanced, not just because we're queer, but because we exclusively bottle fed. Because we were both recovering from post-traumatic stress disorder (PTSD), we split the night, every night.

Will feeling bad emotionally affect my milk?

There's no denying that having a newborn increases the stress levels of everybody involved. Short-term negative feelings won't affect the quality of your milk or milk production in any significant way. If you're particularly stressed during a feeding or pumping session, the milk you produce at that time might have higher levels of cortisol in it but outside a laboratory environment it would be largely undetectable. The milk you make when you're stressed is still what your baby needs and won't make your baby stressed.

If you consistently feel bad when you're feeding or pumping, this may be indicative of a specific hormonal imbalance called *dysphoric milk ejection reflex* (D-MER), which is caused by a sudden drop in dopamine levels when milk release is triggered. This can lead to a sudden feeling of hopelessness, anger, dread, or other feelings associated with depression. There is no specific treatment, but it usually subsides in a few minutes when your oxytocin levels go up. In my experience as a lactation consultant, this is the kind of thing where knowing what's happening and knowing that it is temporary can make the experience more tolerable. Another point to note is that a sudden increase in oxytocin levels during milk release sometimes causes nausea. While this may be uncomfortable, it should pass quickly and is not a cause for alarm without other symptoms (Wambach & Spencer, 2019).

Another point to consider is whether there are outside forces that are contributing to you feeling bad. As AJ explains, if you feel as if something is going wrong, examine why and how heavily you should value that opinion:

> Another one of my favorite staple questions in all circumstances, but this includes lactation, is, "Who told you that?"
> "Oh, but I'm not making enough milk."
> "Who told you that?"
> "The baby is feeding more often."
> Okay, but baby is also six weeks old and what we know about human development around six weeks of age is that baby's gotta feed more.
> "Oh, well. I just don't think my milk is good enough quality."

"Who told you that?"

What we do know about human evolution and mammalian species is that there is a possibility that your milk isn't good enough, but it's so minute that actually, let's deal with the overwhelmingly likely possibility that it's a growth spurt or it's a feeding cue or whatever it might be.

"Who told you that?" can be such a powerful question. A lot of the time, the one who told you that is a patriarchal society that undervalues human lactation.

If you can identify gender dysphoria as the source of your added stress, remember that lactation has less to do with your gender identity and more to do with your identity as a mammal.

As Anissa says:

> For me it was just this cool mammal thing that has nothing to do with womanhood or femininity. It's just like, okay, cool I feel like a gorilla, or a tiger or whatever that's like lactating, being pregnant and stuff. It was kind of the same way with chestfeeding. Just doing the cool mammal thing. It really doesn't have anything to do with gender.

How can I stop producing milk?

Stopping lactation, or *involution*, can be done safely and effectively on your own as long as you don't try to rush it. The most important thing is to gradually remove milk so your body has less to replace. This is simply done by waiting until your chest is uncomfortable with milk, then pumping, hand expressing, or latching your baby *just until the pressure is relieved*. Repeat this for several days until your supply eventually wanes.

If you decide to stop lactating because of gender dysphoria, then you may be relieved to learn that some of the things you do to help feel like yourself may also be effective in involution. As I discuss in the next two questions, it's possible that binding and/or testosterone can decrease the amount of milk you produce, but it's certain that either won't cause higher milk production. If you're looking to speed up the process, over the counter decongestants will also help as well as herbal remedies like mint or sage tea. Basically, if something is good for a runny nose, it's bad for milk production. I would be remiss, however, if I didn't remind you to *always* consult with a doctor before taking any medication for an off-label purpose.

Anissa provided me with a good example of how they prepared a patient for the eventuality of milk production and how to minimize its effect. I hope their words will help you as well:

> His chest had always been an area of dysphoria before he got pregnant and he knew that it was more important to him to have the chest he needed than to be able to nurse. And so with him it was mostly just a matter of letting him know beforehand, like hey your milk is still gonna try to come in so you might have a little bit of swelling, in whatever tissue you do have left, in the armpit and whatnot, the upper chest where the mastectomy doesn't affect as much. So he was prepared for that and knew that it goes away within a few days. We talked about gentle massage, and sage tea as other good ways to decrease the amount of milk, and he did that. The milk went away in under a week and he was fine. But just being prepared for that is important.

For those who need to stop producing milk on a very short timetable, there are two medications available which work by reducing prolactin levels, thereby cutting down milk production. These are *cabergoline* and *bromocriptine*, although they are only available with a prescription.

When can I bind?

In my experience, people who don't have cause to bind or have a lot of experience with people who do tend to not understand the significance and may equate the recommendation (or at times mandate) to not bind as being on par with any recommendation to wear loose-fitting clothing. In fact, for many people, it is about so much more than physical comfort and should be treated accordingly. Victoria offers an excellent assessment of the idea of binding in much of the medical field and how a professional can work past it:

> I think that a lot of our perspective that trans people shouldn't bind in pregnancy and lactation is not evidence-based and there are just ways that I feel like our field limits people's autonomy because we aren't thinking about it broadly enough. I think that the benefits of binding are not fully understood by practitioners in our field. For some people it is really important to them, and postpartum, whether they've had top surgery or not. But if you've had top surgery and you've had regrowth and you're going through a gendered experience postpartum, I want people to have that tool available to them. And so what that looks like to me is teaching someone a lot of lymphatic drainage techniques and empowering someone to be in charge of their own body and notice whether they are having areas of swelling or soreness because of the binder they're using.

In practical terms, you should only start binding when it feels physically comfortable to do so, and I recommend easing back into it. The first few times you bind while lactating, you may want to stay home just to make sure you have an idea of how your body will react. You don't want to be in the middle of the grocery store or driving and suddenly have shooting pain. Start after you have fed your baby or pumped (in other words, when your chest feels empty) and limit binding time to no more than an hour or less initially.

Regarding the lymphatic drainage techniques that Victoria refers to, she writes about them extensively in her own book, *Feed the Baby*, but has also provides us with a brief explanation:

> So the lymphatic drainage massage, it's really simple: it's really, really gentle and you're doing a lot of sort of waking up your lymphatic system with gentle massage directly around the lymph nodes and then encouraging fluid back and out through that system instead of just moving milk forward. Understand that a lot of the discomfort and mastitis and what we perceive as clogged ducts is actually a pattern of inflammation in really tight complex gland tissue.

The specific techniques for lymphatic drainage massage are similar to those I describe for massaging in preparation to induce lactation in Chapter 5. Additionally, you have lymph nodes in your neck and armpits, so gently massaging those places in small circles with your fingertips will also help if you're experiencing pain or inflammation. Even if they don't feel swollen specifically, there will be no downside to the practice. This is especially important if you've ever had any surgeries in these areas, be it a broken bone or something as simple as a mole removal (Facelli, 2023).

There are some risks associated with binding while lactating. Although it should not be considered definite, prolonged compression *can* lead to clogged ducts. In a best-case scenario, these are uncomfortable but can be manually rubbed or worked out using a vibrator, electric toothbrush, or similar item. If unnoticed or left untreated, however, they can become infected and lead to engorgement or mastitis, which may require medical attention. If binding consistently is very important to your mental health but it is negatively impacting your physical health, you might consider suppressing lactation so that you can bind for longer periods of time more safely. All choices are valid, and I support you in doing what's best for your family.

When can I (re)start taking testosterone?

It seems to be a fairly common assumption that if you want to lactate you shouldn't take testosterone. There are some potential "risks" to using testosterone while lactating, but this blanket recommendation is misleading and doesn't make space for nuance. The decision to start or restart using testosterone should be based on how you feel about your body and the amount of milk you are producing. These two factors may hold different priorities for you personally, and you get to decide what you need and want most in order to show up as your best new-parent self.

The reason lactating parents are often discouraged from taking testosterone is that testosterone is thought to inhibit milk production. However, research is showing that it's not consistently working that way. There are stories about parents resuming testosterone and their milk supply decreasing significantly, but it seems to be just as common that milk supply decreases only slightly or not at all. There's very little clinical data on this, but what we do have indicates that we cannot assume how hormone replacement therapy will affect you personally.

For those of you worried that testosterone injections will affect the quality of the milk you are producing, it will not. That is a fact. We have research that shows the amount of testosterone that ends up in your milk is practically zero. Furthermore, testosterone is not absorbed by the stomach very well (which is why we have shots instead of pills), so pretty much all of the testosterone that does end up in the milk will just pass right through your baby. If you find that testosterone is affecting you in unpleasant ways, you can always talk to your provider about stopping again (Oberhelman-Eaton *et al.*, 2021).

On the other hand, if you prefer using testosterone gel to injections, you need to be extremely careful in how and where you apply it to avoid any accidental contact with the baby. Any testosterone gel that gets onto the baby's skin will be absorbed and can cause serious hormonal imbalances.

Does it matter if I've had (or plan to have) top surgery?

This is a big one, and, perhaps frustratingly, the answer is "maybe." If you have already had top surgery, the biggest factor is whether you and your doctor knew ahead of time that lactation might be on the table for you. If you plan ahead for the potential of lactation, the doctor can focus on removing *adipose* (fatty) tissue, while leaving the milk glands and ducts as intact as possible. Even if milk ducts are removed, they are surprisingly good at repairing themselves and regrowing, so you will typically still be able to produce and express *some* milk.

The same goes if you have your nipple repositioned. If it wasn't necessary to reposition the nipple or your doctor intentionally avoided it, then removing milk shouldn't be a problem. If your nipple was regrafted, then milk will still be able to come out, just not as prevalently, and clogged ducts may become a regular part of your lactation journey (West, 2008).

However, professional support will be available, because this is very much like the experience of cis women who give birth and have a condition called *insufficient glandular tissue* (IGT), as Kristin-Cole explains:

> Feeding after surgery is not all that different from feeding with IGT, from a physical standpoint. There's just not glandular tissue, so we're working with other ways to deal with that. And I love supplemental nursing symptoms, they're what made me be able to nurse my kids. I feel really strongly about making sure that people have access to that information. I think a lot of lactation consultants gatekeep supplemental nursing systems because they think they're

too difficult. And I think that they are amazing, and I always tell clients that you will curse me for the first three days but if you stick with it, then you'll love it. And it generally turns out to be true. So with people who've had top surgery and want to chestfeed, that's where we end up going for the most part. It feels like there's so many trans guys having babies, I guess because I'm in a having babies sort of profession. *(Supplemental nursing systems, also called a supplemental feeding device, are discussed in more detail in Chapter 3.)*

If your nipple was removed entirely and there is no outlet for the milk you produce, then lactation should be suppressed as soon as possible. Your body will stop producing milk once it realizes that none is being removed, but there are medications (both prescription and over-the-counter) available to speed the process along, and cold pads can be used to aid swelling. This is definitely a situation where I would recommend seeing an IBCLC or other medical professional, if possible, just to make sure you don't have any major problems as you begin involution.

If you plan to have top surgery but believe you might want to produce milk for future offspring, make certain your doctor knows about your decision and keep in mind that this will probably have a strong bearing on any decisions made concerning your nipple and areola size and placement.

Does lactating keep me from menstruating?

Lactational amenorrhea, or not menstruating while you're lactating, is an evolutionary advantage that prevents humans from becoming pregnant while they already have a newborn. I'm sure that on the whole this has been a widely successful evolutionary feature, but it cannot be considered a sure thing. Generally speaking, you only have a 1–2% chance of becoming pregnant if all of the following three things are true: you are currently amenorrheic *and* the baby is getting all or nearly all of their calories from your milk *and* the baby is less than six months old. The six-month point is added because that's often when people start adding complementary foods, but studies have shown that the system may hold true for up to 12 months if the first two criteria are still met (Berens & Labbok, 2015). In 1998, the World Health Organization did an international study of 4118 dyads in seven countries to determine the main factors in how long the effect lasts and found that the more time a baby stays latched in the course of a day and the percentage of the infant's calories that come from milk are the main contributing factors related to feeding. The number of times the parent has given birth and the number of times the baby has had to be treated for illness are additional factors contributing to longer amenorrhea.

If birth control while lactating is your goal, hormonal birth control, either progestin only or in combination with estrogen, has the highest chance of interrupting your milk supply, especially if started before lactation is well established. For temporary birth control, you're better off going with barriers (condoms or a diaphragm). Emergency contraceptive pills may impact lactation in the short term, and so the progestin-only variety (Plan B) is preferred but we have no reason to believe that any will be detrimental to lactation in the long term (Berens & Labbok, 2015).

What if I get pregnant?

Lactational amenorrhea is not a sure-fire method of birth control, especially after your baby is six months old. There's a fairly common misconception that if you become pregnant while you're still lactating, you either will automatically stop making milk or you should intentionally stop making milk for the good of the new fetus. Neither of these is true; however, you will probably produce less milk and the consistency and/or flavor of your milk often changes, leading the older child to choose to wean.

If you're lactating while pregnant, your daily water and caloric needs will be rather high, so make sure you're eating enough and drinking enough water. Uterine contractions are also to be expected. However, although there is not much clinical research on the matter, preterm labor is not considered a significant risk.

After you have the new baby, your older child may have a renewed interest in your milk, chest or nipples and want to feed along with their new sibling. As long as the younger child is having first crack at each side, there is no reason not to let the elder finish up, as it were. Since we know milk production is based on how much is being removed, this will help ensure you have a good supply.

Can I make milk for the baby I'm adopting?

You can! There are a lot of options for the exact process you might want to use and a lot of factors determining how long it will take. So many that Chapters 4–8 are entirely devoted to *inducing lactation*.

CHAPTER 3

What's a Non-Lactating Parent to Do?

This chapter is a slightly edited re-print of an article that appeared in the Spring/Summer 2021 edition of *Everyday Birth Magazine*. It is worth mentioning that all of this information, particularly the notes I added at the end, also applies to parents whose partners are inducing lactation even if they are not yet making milk.

So your partner or your surrogate just gave birth, or your adoption just went through, you just started fostering an infant, or you ended up with a baby by one of the myriad other ways people do. But you have a baby now, and you're not lactating. And more to the point, you don't *want* to be lactating.

Maybe someone else in the family is making milk, but feeding your baby doesn't need to be just one person's job and you've got so much bonding to do! Maybe nobody's making milk and all the parents can use this information. Bottle feeding is the usual answer, but did you know there are a few other ways to get milk or formula into your little bub? Talk to a lactation consultant before trying any of these, just to make sure you're doing it right.

- *Supplemental feeding device (SFD).* These have a variety of names depending on the brand, but they all use the word supplemental or supplementer. This method encourages maximum bonding because your baby is suckling your nipple just as if you were lactating, but the food comes from a feeding tube snuck into the corner of your baby's mouth. The other end of the tube is in either a bottle, pouch or a feeding syringe. If this sounds a bit complex, that's because it is and it can definitely take a while to get the hang of it. So why bother? Aside from the aforementioned bonding that comes with holding a baby close as they learn to associate your body with warmth and comfort, this method is particularly good for parents who are trying to induce lactation or relactate. No pump in the world will stimulate milk flow as effectively as an actual hungry baby.

- *Finger feeding.* This method is similar to an SFD except that the feeding tube is taped to a person's finger instead of near the nipple. This technique is rarely used long term, but it's included here because parents using an SFD may need to switch from time to time and it's useful for people to have as many options as possible.

  The basic idea is that your baby thinks the finger is a nipple and as they suck they get the milk or formula which is being slowly pushed through a feeding syringe. As with SFD feeding, the technique can be tricky. Hands need to be extremely clean and fingernails trimmed short. A healthcare provider doing this should have gloves on, but parents doing it daily might decide against gloves.

  You insert your finger nail-side down to keep it away from the soft palate. If you go too far in you can make your baby gag and might need to calm them before you try again. If your baby doesn't open their mouth on their own, gently touching their top lip will usually cause them to reflexively open wide. As soon as you feel the wave-motion of their tongue, either you or someone else can start slowly depressing the plunger on the feeding syringe. They also make syringes for this purpose that have a curved tip, so you can bypass the feeding tube entirely. It can take a while to get the hang of; but this technique is particularly good if you're already doing SFD and someone unfamiliar needs to feed your baby or if your baby is brand new and having trouble feeding, either because of a weak suck or they are having trouble coordinating sucking and breathing. In either case, you will almost certainly have seen a lactation consultant before using this technique.

- *Spoon or cup feeding.* Think of it like using a sippy cup for people who are too small to do it on their own. Like the previous method, this is rarely done long term but can be very helpful when you're avoiding bottles, or your baby has trouble feeding from a bottle. Basically, what you're doing is allowing your baby to drink from either a small cup (think medicine cup or egg cup) or a regular spoon but instead of pouring milk into your baby's mouth it's more like a kitten lapping up milk with the tip of their tongue. There is also a device historically used with preterm babies in India called a *paladai* that works on a similar principle.

What if your baby is exclusively feeding at the chest and pumped milk is going straight into the freezer for later use? If a lactating parent wants to do this and it's working well, the best thing you can do is to support them. How can you do this? So glad you asked:

- *Help during the day.* I tell people that the first step to being helpful is to say, "What can I do to be helpful?" But if you're looking for ideas, some good ones are: making sure the comfy space on the couch is clear and clean, keeping snacks and water nearby, and keeping track of how long your baby ate and on which side (this can go from helpful to annoying really quickly, so be sure to communicate if it's actually helpful or feeling micromanage-y).

- *Keep track of output.* I'm not saying that only one parent should be responsible for changing diapers, but it is a good idea to have one parent who is responsible for knowing how many wet and bowel movement (BM) diapers there are on a day-to-day basis. Since there's no way to know exactly how much liquid is going into an exclusively chestfeeding baby, it's worth keeping track of approximately how much is coming out of them. Since this will vary by age and weight, check with your pediatrician or lactation consultant for how many wet and BM diapers your baby is expected to have every day or week.

- *Be the first one up at night.* Sometimes when a baby wakes up at night it means they're hungry; but sometimes they're gassy, or startled, or accidentally poked themselves in the eye. If a non-lactating parent gets in the habit of being the first one up when your baby cries and only wakes up the lactating parent if your baby shows signs of hunger, then they can help maximize rest for the parent who is probably spending the most time with your baby when the sun is up. What are signs of hunger? The most common ones are turning the head to one side (also called *rooting*), lip smacking, and chewing on their cute little fist.

Since writing this chapter, I have a few more items I would add to the list of how you can support lactating parents:

- *Read everything your partner wants you to.* You probably don't both need to read the entirety of *What to Expect...* (Murkoff, 2024) or *Feed the Baby* (Facelli, 2023), but if there are certain sections your partner thinks are important, make sure to take that seriously. Only you know how much time you have available to add things to your reading list, so do this to the best of your ability and see if you can get help prioritizing what to read if you're feeling overwhelmed. Alternatively, you could also be the first to read some of the books and sort out which information will be most relevant to your family. This suggestion also applies to websites, podcasts, and that sort of thing. If your partner asks you to give it a listen, what could it hurt?

- *Find help before you need it.* Another way you can be helpful is to proactively find out if there are any queer or queer-competent lactation consultants local to you. For most lactation difficulties and questions, a telehealth consultation will suffice so you will have a much broader search area. However, if there is a difficulty where a physical examination is necessary (usually if there are concerns about the baby's oral anatomy), then having someone ready to turn to will pay dividends. The last thing you want is for both of you to be sleep deprived and your baby to be underfed, and you trying to find a medical professional who won't create a whole new set of problems. Furthermore, depending on where you live, your medical insurance may cover your lactation care with certain providers. So if you're lucky, you can have someone lined up who will provide the care your family needs, and it won't cost you an arm and a leg.

PART 2

HOW TO MAKE MILK WITHOUT BEING PREGNANT

CHAPTER 4

Inducing Lactation

I can't count the number of times I've told people how they can make milk without ever being pregnant, only to have them respond with something to the effect of, "I wish I'd known about this five years ago when my wife gave birth!" or, "I wish somebody had told me that when I was adopting!" While it seems that almost all lactation consultants know that this is an option, getting the word out to the people who might benefit the most from this information has proved trying.

There are several reasons a person may choose to lactate regardless of whether they can gestate a child. Apart from all the well-known benefits of human milk and bodyfeeding discussed throughout this book, a non-gestational parent might choose to induce lactation as a way to feel emotionally closer to the baby, assert their own feelings of parenthood, gender euphoria, or just for the unique experience of it. After all, how many times in your life will this opportunity present itself?

Generally speaking, femme identified people (trans or cis) are those most interested in inducing, although there is no reason to exclude from this discussion nonbinary and trans masculine people who are also interested in making milk. Cis men occasionally seek me out with questions about inducing lactation, and often start taking birth control and/or domperidone while pumping, but in my personal experience none has ever produced milk. I have talked with other consultants who have had cis men produce milk, and there are documented reports of this (Diamond, 1997) which I talk about later in the book, for interested parties. While the details will vary based on the individual, the overall process of inducing lactation is generally the same regardless of your current gender or any other gender you may have been assigned or identify as.

Resources on inducing lactation generally rely on specific procedures or protocols, with the Newman-Goldfarb Protocol (developed by Drs. Lenore Goldfarb and Jack Newman, 2002) being the most well known and established, along with the Three Step Framework for Inducing Lactation (designed by Alyssa Schnell, 2022). Both of these are very user friendly and not written in an over-medicalized way so as to be accessible for parents interested in trying. The Newman-Goldfarb does assume that you are a cis woman who is not taking any sort of hormone treatment, which can lead to difficulties when you get to the part about taking birth control pills.

Schnell's Framework makes fewer assumptions about the patient and seems to be specifically designed with the knowledge that all people are different, but it is written for professionals as opposed to parents, so finding it takes a little more digging if you don't have easy access to the *Journal of Human Lactation*. It is also available through her website, in a course designed for lactation professionals.

Although there are differences and variations, both of these are essentially divided into three steps: preparing your body to make milk, expressing milk to be collected before the baby arrives, and increasing your supply as you feed your new baby.

To me, the problem with this approach is that it assumes things like considering and discussing your goals are implied, or that everyone will have the same lactation goals, which isn't a reasonable expectation. I think lactation professionals forget that people don't know what they don't know, and we should not count on patients to have expectations if they have no lactation experience. Therefore, in Chapter 5, I've added discussing expectations and setting goals as a new Step 1, which is then revisited in between each of the other three steps listed above.

I will be the first to admit that the procedure set out in Chapter 5 is not very different from either the Newman-Goldfarb Protocol or Schnell's Framework, and these extra steps can be incorporated into either of those. I just feel that lactation professionals should not be underselling the value of talking things through.

The Steps

Step 1: Form a plan, set goals and expectations

Before you even need to think about the details of preparing your body to start making milk, it's prudent to consider what your goals are, what you're willing to do to meet those goals, and what you'll do if you can't meet them. The good news is that by picking up this or any other book on lactation, you've already started! The questions that follow are important to ask yourself now and periodically throughout your lactation journey. If the baby will have any parents besides yourself, it's important to involve them in this as well. Any lactation consultant will tell you that support from their partners is one of the key factors in people accomplishing their lactation goals.

Here, AJ shares some of their experience with two sets of parents inducing lactation who have very different strategies and goals, reminding us that there is no single correct strategy:

> I've worked with two different trans women who have induced lactation. The gestational parent was a nonbinary person in the first family I worked with. They were 12 weeks pregnant when I started working with them so she was already well underway in her inducing lactation journey, as was the second family. I think she was about five or six months pregnant. She was quite a bit further on than the

first family, but yeah, I still spoke to them about their process and what they had been doing up until now so that I could be informed about when they were going to dump their estrogen and up their pumping routine or whatever it might have been. I'm very much involved with the non-gestational parent because they're the best placed person to support the gestational parent. So let's support them to do their jobs as well.

The last family I worked with, she took everything. If she read a book, study, or whatever, and there was something that said that it had any effect on lactation, she took it. She used to joke, "If you shake me I'll rattle." But the first family I worked with, she was very much more just wanting to be able to calm the baby. She wasn't really worried about how much she made. Whereas, you know, completely the opposite end of the spectrum for the second woman I've worked with inducing lactation—she had a spreadsheet and everything.

People are different in how they learn and what they perceive are the signs that lactation is going well, that the infant feeding journey is going well. For the second woman I worked with, she wanted to see it all on the spreadsheet and for the first, she wanted to see the baby fall asleep at her breast, that was all she wanted. I mean, they had very different requirements, very different goals, for their induction of lactation.

One of the things I've talked about in my workshop is please just talk to your clients, your service users, about their goals. Because with the first woman, if I'd gone bowling in saying, "Right, you need to get on the Newman-Goldfarb and you need to start power pumping..." that was all pointless. That could have been time that we spent bonding and talking to each other, supporting the gestational parent, loving the unit as a whole, you know, and talking about ways in which to encourage baby to latch. Like learning an SNS (supplemental nursing system), you know, having a go at that and getting some time doing other things to promote oxytocin and bonding rather than worrying about writing down all the medications. Because it wasn't going to be strictly necessary for her goal to be able to do that.

Have you ever lactated or been pregnant in the past?

The answer to this question will probably not change while you are in the process of inducing lactation, but many clients don't realize how relevant it is when they are first weighing their options. There is no consensus on exactly how long glandular changes last after pregnancy or lactation, but if the last time you lactated was within about three years, it might be more accurate to refer to what you're planning as *relactation*.

Sometimes people begin a bodyfeeding relationship but have to stop early for reasons beyond their control (often an unforeseen medical event), then decide they want to start again a few months later. Sometimes people give birth to a baby and have a chestfeeding relationship, then some time later their partner becomes pregnant and they decide to lactate again. These are both examples of relactation. There's no strict definition for when you are relactating as opposed to inducing lactation, but suffice to say that if it's been less than three years since the last time you produced milk you'll almost certainly have a faster time than someone who has never produced milk. If you still find yourself leaking periodically (as sometimes happens when a person is aroused or hears a crying baby), the process will probably be easier still.

Are you interested in taking medications to induce?

To be extremely clear, unless you are a cis man, I would never say that a patient would be *required* to take medication in order to produce milk. Even in that case, there is reason to believe it's not 100% necessary, which I discuss in Appendix B. For everybody else, depending on your individual body and medical history, pumping and massaging alone may be sufficient to produce milk. If you are interested in adding medications to your regimen, consult with your primary doctor before starting anything new as there may be drug interactions you're unaware of. Details about some of the medications people commonly use to induce lactation, including other professional's opinions on their necessity, are discussed in Step 2.

Are you interested in taking herbal or dietary supplements?

As with medications, there are also pros and cons to taking herbal supplements. To me the biggest con is inconsistent regulation, meaning that, if you do decide to take any, it can be difficult to know the quality and amount of the active compounds. The concern about drug interactions also exists with supplements, so be sure to double check any herbs you want to take against any medications you currently are taking.

Most of the herbs associated with lactation don't have clinical research backing them up, but it's important to remember that the placebo effect is absolutely real. If your friends and family are convinced something is going to help you, you might as well consider trying it. More extensive information on *galactagogues*, or milk-producing foods and herbs are found in Tables 5.1 and 5.2.

If you aren't sure what you want to take, but feel as if you should start doing *something*, start taking a prenatal vitamin. There is no reason not to take them if you're a healthy person with no dietary restrictions, and the extra vitamins and minerals that benefit pregnant people are the same that lactating people need. I pretty much always recommend my patients begin taking prenatal vitamins, or continue if they already have been taking them.

Do you have a date you'd like to be producing milk by?

If you have a specific due date for your baby, you'll be able to better manage your plan. I usually recommend people start their process at the beginning of the second trimester, if possible. However, for many, this is simply not possible. If you're in a situation where you

Table 5.1: Food galactagogues

Food galacta-gogues	What is it?	Might it work?	Is it harmful?
Anise	Commonly used cooking herb.	Widely used as a galacta-gogue in small doses, little clinical evidence.	In large doses may hinder milk production and contains chemicals which may be adverse to infants.
Basil	Commonly used cooking herb.	Historical precedent but should not be taken in large doses.	Fresh basil is fine when used as a food or spice. Supplemental use is discouraged when pregnant or lactating.
Beer	Beverage with an alcohol content of 3–10%	People think of beer as a galactagogue because it is made with hops and barley, is calorie dense, and helps you relax. For these reasons, it may help.	The alcohol content inhibits milk production, so I wouldn't recommend it as a galactagogue. See Chapter 11 for more information on drinking alcohol while making milk.
Fennel	The seed is a common cooking spice, the plant itself is eaten cooked or raw.	Historical precedent exists but no clinical research.	Apart from people with allergies, there is no reason to think fennel may be harmful.
Fenu-greek	Cooking spice.	If you take large amounts (3500–7000 mg/day).	Do not take if you are allergic to chickpeas or peanuts, have diabetes or any blood disorders.
Garlic	Cooking spice.	Historical precedent but no clinical research.	No.
Grains (oats, barley, millet, etc.)	Food.	Historical precedent but no clinical research.	You probably eat a lot of grains anyway. There's no real downside to eating more but it probably won't help.
Hops	Herb used in beer brewing.	Historical precedent but no clinical research.	Some of the estrogenic compounds in hops may cause a decrease in milk production.
Seaweed	Various seaweeds are foods in many countries.	Seaweed works as a galactagogue if your diet is otherwise low in iodine.	You could potentially end up with too much iodine if you eat excessive amounts.

(Brodribb, 2018; Ruddle, 2020; Schnell, 2013)

Table 5.2: Herbal galactagogues

Herbal galactagogue	What is it?	Might it work?	Is it harmful?
Alfalfa	Also called *lucerne*. A plant commonly used as animal feed but has medicinal properties.	Supports function of the pituitary gland, which controls prolactin and oxytocin.	Alfalfa is a legume, so people allergic to chickpeas or peanuts should steer clear.
Brewer's yeast	Yeast used to make beer, actually a fungus.	Included in a lot of lactation cookie recipes. It will probably help because it's high in B vitamins.	Avoid it if you are prone to yeast infections or fungal infections.
Dandelion	Leaves are used as a food; root and leaves are dried as a medicinal herb.	Historical precedent but no clinical research supporting use.	Taken as a supplement, dandelion is a diuretic so may cause dehydration. Avoid large doses.
Goat's rue	Medicinal herb.	A phytoestrogen which behaves like estrogen in the body. It may help people start making milk.	If you are already making milk, the phytoestrogens will not increase your supply and may be detrimental.
Marshmallow	Medicinal herb.	Historical precedent but no clinical research supporting use.	It does seem to be generally good for you, with no downside to taking it.
Milk thistle	Medicinal herb also called *blessed thistle*.	Historical precedent and some clinical research supporting use.	Do not use it if you are allergic to ragweed, daisies, chrysanthemums, or marigolds. Use caution if you are taking antipsychotics, blood thinners or medication for seizures, anxiety, or cancer.
Moringa	Food and medicinal herb in many Asian countries. Also called *malunggay*.	Extremely nutrient-dense. Will probably help when eaten or taken as a supplement. Some clinical research shows an increase in milk production.	If taking dried as a supplement, do not take beyond recommended dosages.
Saw palmetto	Medicinal herb.	Has lots of fatty acids, which may increase milk production.	Some studies indicate it may cause hormonal imbalances.
Shatavari	Medicinal herb.	Historical precedent for use in lactation. Lots of medicinal uses, generally considered "good for you."	Couldn't hurt when taken moderately. Avoid it if you are allergic to asparagus.
Torbangun	Medicinal herb.	May help activate milk ducts when inducing lactation.	May cause problems with the thyroid gland and cause particular harm to pregnant people.

could have a baby in either two months or two years, you should ask yourself, "Would I rather be pumping for two years, or not start producing milk until after the baby comes?" This is a personal decision and neither of those choices is right or wrong.

How much time per day are you able to devote to pumping/massaging?

The conventional wisdom is that massaging or pumping should be done for a minimum of 20 minutes per side, eight times per day with no more than a six-hour break at night. This is a very fair assessment, and in some cases, more may be needed. If you're using a hand pump or hand expressing, this will change to five hours and 20 minutes per day. If that sounds like too big a time commitment, you may want to invest in a double-electric pump which can do both sides simultaneously, and this will bring the total to two hours and 40 minutes per day. There are many other factors to consider and there is a more thorough discussion on pumps in Chapter 6.

How much milk do you want to be making?

Are you hoping to make all the milk your child needs or would you be thrilled to make any milk at all? Again, this is a personal question which has no correct or incorrect answer, and in fact you may find your answer changes over the course of your journey. Bear in mind that if there will be another lactating parent, you will likely both need to maintain a pumping schedule in order to ensure that enough milk is being removed to maintain your supplies.

What will you do if you can't make as much as you had hoped?

Given the unpredictability of individual bodies in the process of inducing lactation, it's worthwhile to consider not only what your goals are but also what you will do if you can't accomplish those goals.

Right now, you have no way of knowing how much milk you will be able to produce, but if your goal is to provide all the milk for your baby and later on it starts to look as if that won't be possible, you should consider in advance if you want to begin sourcing human milk from other people or if formula would be best for you and your family. Maybe right now you think that you'll never give the baby formula, but after you spend a few months thinking about it, you might become more comfortable with the idea.

Are there any lactation consultants local to you who are competent in working with your needs and demographics?

You don't necessarily *need* a lactation consultant to successfully induce lactation, either of the protocols discussed previously can be found online and there are many other books and communities available, but at some point on your journey you may decide to seek out professional guidance and it's good to know ahead of time who specifically you should be talking to.

Don't fret if there aren't any people locally, you probably won't need an in-person consultation for information on inducing; most of my consultations are phone calls with people who are either interested in learning more about the process or are already pumping and just have a few questions. However, if you do decide to find someone you can see in person, make sure that they are experienced or at least educated in inducing lactation specifically. Lactation education is incredibly varied, so while most consultants know a little something about inducing, most have not actually helped someone induce. How much experience or training you're looking for in a consultant is up to you, and you may need to balance it with other factors, such as cultural competence and experience working with (or being a member of) the queer or transgender community. Coral, whose full story is included in Chapter 8, shares her experience working with an IBCLC experienced in inducing but not working in the trans community:

I think I was like the first trans woman she had ever talked to.

So it would have been helpful to work with someone who knew anything about trans people. She's like, really sweet, and has tried to be really helpful and she *has* been helpful in lots of ways. But there's just like, a lot of pretty basic things about how my body works that she didn't really understand. She definitely expected my body to work in the same way that a cis woman's body would work. So it's a little bit challenging and clunky. But I appreciate the things that she was helpful with.

Step 2: Prepare your body to make milk

While you may not have total control over when your body starts to make milk or when your baby will arrive, the choice of when to begin preparing your body starts largely when you say it does (supply chains and work schedules notwithstanding).

If you're feeling ambitious, Step 2 can potentially start on the same day as Step 1 and last until your body begins making milk, possibly six-to-eight weeks or maybe longer. If you decide to take birth control in order to simulate pregnancy, an ideal situation would be for you to start about 24 weeks before the baby's due date. This will allow 16 weeks for the hormones to do their thing and will acclimate your body to the new schedule, plus eight weeks of pumping, which should afford enough time to start producing milk. This is by no means required though, and many people just start pumping and eventually produce milk.

Medications

Keep taking any medications and supplements you have been, unless they are known to hinder lactation (there is a discussion of which medications are contraindicated for lactation in Chapter 11). For the most part, now isn't the time to make any additional changes to your routine. In terms of adding medications, consider the following aspects.

Hormones (Birth control pills)

If you aren't already taking hormone treatments and you have a few months of lead time, you will increase your chance of making milk if you can convince your body that you are pregnant. For most people, regardless of currently having or having ever had a uterus and/or ovaries, the convenient way to do this is by taking estrogen and progesterone in the form of combination birth control pills. It's worth considering that these can also cause emotional or mood changes, which you may consider drawbacks or even deal breakers (Skovlund *et al.*, 2016). While this will almost certainly speed up your milk production start time, it is not 100% necessary if taking hormones is not something you're comfortable with or you're unable to get them.

If you've already been taking birth control pills for their intended purpose, you've done that bit and you just need to stop taking them. In this case, you may want to start a new form of birth control for the time being. If you're new to birth control pills, you don't need to take them for the full 40 weeks—12 or 16 is often sufficient. Be sure to skip the non-hormonal pills (often called the *sugar pills*) in the packet. After three or four months, you'll want to stop taking them and, within 24 hours, begin your pumping regimen as though you have just had a newborn baby. As discussed in Chapter 9, estrogen and progesterone get the ball rolling for lactation, but inhibit milk production, which is why pregnant people don't usually start lactating until after they give birth.

People who are already receiving estrogen and/or progesterone treatments (or any other hormone therapy) may be able to skip this, but will probably need to make changes to their dosages and should definitely talk to their prescribing doctors or a lactation professional before making any changes.

Rebekah, a lactation consultant with both personal and professional experience of inducing, has had mixed results with patients who have not taken birth control and just started pumping and taking domperidone or herbs:

> I have definitely worked with parents who, for one reason or another, don't want to use the medications: they are uncomfortable with them or their doctor isn't comfortable with them, or they have some sort of health thing that interferes with taking any of the medications.
>
> I've definitely worked with parents that are inducing and attempting with just pumping or can't take birth control and so they're just pumping and taking domperidone. I would say that pumping and domperidone is hit or miss, a lot of people can get a good amount of milk but not 25–30 ounces.
>
> In my experience with just pumping and galactagogues or herbs, they rarely reach a full supply of milk unless they have previously lactated. I know there are some really rare cases that I've talked with, but I think for the most part they usually get some milk after months of pumping. But I've had a parent who pumped for six months and was still just getting drops on pumping and herbs and so that's definitely something. When someone comes to consult with me, I am very honest upfront.

Domperidone (Motilium)

So what is this domperidone that everybody's using to induce lactation? Domperidone (sold under the brand name Motilium) is actually a gastrointestinal medication that has a side effect of increasing prolactin levels and thereby causing milk production. Since its legality varies from country to country, depending on where you live, it will either be fairly common and easy to get or you may have to find a way to order it online. People's experience with domperidone varies, but most people have no unpleasant side effects. There are studies that show domperidone can cause *cardiac arrhythmia* (or irregular heartbeat), which is especially noteworthy if you were assigned male at birth, because we are more likely to have heart problems as we age; but this is very rare when it's taken orally (as opposed to intravenously) by healthy people. There are also less commonly reported side effects, which I learned about while interviewing Rebekah:

> I think the main side effect I had, which I know is what a lot of people are concerned about, is weight gain. I did gain like 30 pounds. I know a lot of people talk when they're on domperidone that they gain steadily over time. But I had a kind of thing where for the first year I was on it I didn't gain at all and then suddenly I hit 13 months on it and I gained, like, 20 pounds in a month, which was very strange. But since then I've talked to other moms on domperidone and literally the exact same thing happened.

It is *extremely important* to note that if someone wants to stop taking domperidone or is not confident in their ability to get more, they should wean themselves off of it. Stopping suddenly can cause withdrawal symptoms, including elevated heart rate, anxiety, and insomnia—and a sudden decrease in milk supply.

Metoclopramide (Reglan)

Like domperidone, metoclopramide (sold under the brand name Reglan) was originally made for problems of the stomach and esophagus and has a side effect of increasing prolactin. Unlike domperidone, while metoclopramide does also encourage milk production, it can also have severe neurological side effects, including depression and *tardive dyskinesia*, which causes uncontrollable movement of the face and arms. Since preparing for and having a new baby can be such an emotionally fraught time to begin with, I steer people away from this medication (Wambach & Spencer, 2019).

None of the above?
Some people aren't comfortable taking medications in general and don't consider inducing lactation a good reason to start. Often, they will double-down on herbal galactagogues, which can work just as well. Victoria talks about her experience as a lactation consultant working with people who chose to mix and match between birth control, herbs, and medications in ways to suit their unique needs:

> I've also had people who just didn't do any of the hormones of the protocol. Or didn't do any of the galactagogues. And that's another spot where it's like, where's your benefit, what is it exactly that you're after? Because sometimes you're wanting some of that experience, which people with low production also have, where you can nurse with very low production and that will work just fine. And so you're after the nursing experience versus the milk production experience; we can manipulate that. And you can do more or less of those protocols as you please. It doesn't need to be an all or nothing.

> And then the other part of this that I think people underestimate, that my mentor Ellen Chetwynd wrote an interesting paper about, is the supply and demand aspect. I don't feel like anybody wants to spend their entire postpartum pumping. So we need to be thinking, okay, what is the overall milk production in this family if there's more than one person producing milk and not more than one baby eating? And so how are you balancing those things so that it's not the case that someone's always pumping while someone's always nursing, unless that really works for you. And babies also sometimes have flow preferences, right? Now that we have more and better supplemental nursing systems on the market, are there options that work well for a family?

> I have not had anyone come to a totally full production with *only* pumping but I've definitely had people go up to full production, wean down off the domperidone and maintain a full production. But I think for some people, the happy medium is the right thing

for their body and family to just pump and not do the hormonal protocols.

And that's sort of part of my stance on lactation in general; we have this kind of exclusivity, all or nothing mentality and we don't have to. I know people who had severe IGT and very, very low production and breastfed for a year and a half while giving bottles of formula. And that was really gender affirming for them. So like, we get to mix and match and we don't have to be all or nothing with this stuff. I think queer people are maybe even a little better at that.

Massaging

The other way to prepare your body is to begin massaging your chest and going through the motions of hand expression at regular intervals throughout the day. This will be beneficial for both physical reasons and psychological ones, especially if your chest is an area you have been uncomfortable with in the past. You can begin this as early as you like, but I usually recommend starting during the second trimester, if possible.

Anything you can do to help acclimate your body to increased contact and prevent yourself from getting "touched out" over the next several months will be remarkably helpful for your mental health and likelihood of success. You can start with three or four 20-minute pumping or massage sessions, which is just first thing in the morning, last thing at night, and then one or two times during the day, and gradually build up to eight sessions in total. You don't have to worry about the six-hour break rule yet. I want to stress the idea that all you're doing is getting your body used to being touched a lot more than usual. This is the time to experiment with how much touching you can stand before it impacts your day-to-day life. Part of the benefit of doing it this way is that you can scale back as needed.

Once you're comfortable with touching your chest several times throughout the day, you can then replace massage sessions with pumping. In this way, you should be less likely to burn out than if you just start pumping eight times per day, although some people take that approach and it works just fine. After a few weeks of consistent massage or pumping, you may start to feel changes in both the tissue itself and your sensitivity. You may even experience some modest growth. This is all very heartening; your body is getting ready to make milk! It's important to note that you probably won't be producing any milk until after you've been mostly pumping consistently for a few weeks. This isn't a rule, though; every person is different. If easing into massaging feels superfluous, you can start pumping as soon as you stop taking birth control.

There are a few different methods for chest massaging, but they all involve gently rubbing your chest in small circles with your fingertips, beginning a few inches outward from the nipple and moving inward. Beyond that, it's just a matter of what is comfortable and works well for you. If you want to use some sort of lubricant, go with a food-type oil like olive or coconut, especially after you start producing milk. You can also use this in your pump flanges, if you have a good fit but feel a little sore.

Pumping

You can start replacing massage sessions with pumping as early as you like and, in theory, never have to switch to a pump if you don't want to or you're producing milk without. The big advantage to pumping is that you can do both sides at the same time, so 40 minutes of massaging becomes 20 minutes of pumping. If you started taking hormones and haven't stopped yet, this is when you'll definitely want to. Rebekah shares her experience as both a parent and a professional with the problem of getting "touched out":

> I would say, if possible, when you're doing the full protocol, pump eight times a day right off the start. I think that is ideal, but I also think if you're not doing the full protocol and you're just starting

pumping and domperidone and not having the birth control involved, I would probably recommend you do it very differently because you can actually get touched out easily. I know parents definitely struggle with pumping and don't enjoy it. I never minded it, which I think is one reason I just ended up doing it for so long. It wasn't really something I minded except for carrying the pump everywhere.

Partner support

If you have a romantic and/or sexual partner, it may only be a matter of time before the fact that you're spending hours a day rubbing your chest or nipples becomes the subject of conversation. When people ask about their partners taking part in the messaging, pumping, or other means of milk removal, what they're often really asking is, "Is it okay for this to feel sexy?" The answer to which is the same answer queer people have been giving to similar questions since the beginning of time: whatever consenting adults are getting up to is no one else's business. Honestly, anything that makes the regular pumping and massaging more enjoyable is a boon. You are dealing with a real live human being here though, which can add a whole new schedule and set of emotions to the equation.

Step 2.5: Consider your goals and expectations again

At some point after you have begun pumping or expressing eight times per day, whether or not you're producing any milk yet, you should revisit your list of questions about goals and expectations. If you're experiencing a lot of growth and increased sensitivity or already producing some milk, you may choose to maintain or increase your expectations; if you feel as if not much is happening, you might want to increase your pumping schedule to see if that helps. It may also be prudent to contact a lactation consultant and discuss other options for when the baby arrives, such as a supplemental feeding device, which you can find an explanation of in Chapter 3.

Pumping is often considered the most important part to successfully inducing, so how do you feel about your schedule? If you're not producing any milk yet, are you experiencing other changes in size, feeling, or sensitivity? Are you having an easy time keeping up with your schedule? Remember that pumping eight times a day is a minimum but it isn't forever, and once the baby arrives you'll be replacing pumping sessions with feeding your baby! If you're having a hard time producing milk you may want to see if you're able to add one or two pumping sessions a day and see if that helps.

Look again at the questions in Step 1, to see if any of your answers have changed.

Step 3: Begin making milk

Step 3 starts when your body begins making milk, so, while you do have a certain amount of control over when that happens, it's not something you can write into your day planner. The first milk to be produced is usually clear or yellowish in color, which people often mistake for colostrum. Colostrum is only made when there has been a placenta so that's not quite correct, but make no mistake that this is milk regardless of the color. Even if it's just a few drops, you can collect it in a feeding syringe, freeze it, label it with the date, and save it for when the baby arrives.

If you haven't started any pumping but have begun making milk while you're doing hand expression, now would be a good time to prioritize trying out a pump. If you find that you're producing more milk with hand expression than pumping, you don't have to switch totally or at all. It's perfectly fine to alternate between hand expressing and pumping throughout the day, if you wish. Ultimately, you want to be either pumping or hand expressing eight times per day in the way that maximizes comfort and milk output for you.

Step 3.5: Once again, consider your goals and expectations

Depending on how things go with the massaging and pumping, you may need to, once again, re-evaluate what your goals are. Maybe instead of producing a full supply, producing half the baby's milk is a more reasonable expectation, especially if you are on a timeline. Remember that even attempting to induce lactation is an exceptional feat and the supply increases slowly when inducing. When the baby arrives and you can feed them directly instead of using the pump, milk may be more forthcoming, but there is rarely the sudden onset of milk that happens when a person gives birth. Even though you can't know how much your baby removes per feeding, you are almost certainly producing more milk when a baby is latched.

Step 4: Maintain or increase your supply

Step 4 begins when you settle into a routine of pumping or hand expressing eight times per day, and hopefully you're removing some amount of milk at each session. Congratulations! Now you are considered to have a supply of milk and your goal shifts to either maintaining or increasing your supply.

The general process for this can be described as more of the same. Increases in the volume of milk made when inducing is usually slow, but steady. I encourage people to keep track of how much milk they're producing, but to do so by recording how many milliliters they produce *daily*. There are too many variables in play for the amount being produced at each session to be significant, and the initial amount of milk is so small that the numbers are perhaps more likely to be discouraging. You might also want to have a daily record of the total, but chart it on a graph as a weekly total (if you're the kind of person who makes a graph). This way, the increases will be more encouraging, but you'll still have an idea of how things are going day-to-day. Once the baby arrives, we can no longer know exactly how much milk is being produced, but as long as the baby is sated and healthy, it's enough. If you aren't producing enough milk to feed the baby exclusively by time they arrive, I recommend feeding them the milk you had frozen earlier using a supplemental feeding device. This way the baby will encourage milk production by being latched, but you can also make sure they're getting enough calories.

As long as you keep up your pumping/feeding schedule, your supply should slowly but surely increase over time.

CHAPTER 6

FAQs about Inducing Lactation

What if I've had (or want to have) implants or a reduction?

Any kind of chest surgery has a chance to negatively impact lactation, especially if it involves removal and regrafting of the nipple-areolar complex (NAC), but there are various factors which will contribute to how big an impact your specific surgery may have.

Implants

For some people, hormones alone are not enough to produce the desired amount of chest tissue to make a person feel affirmed in their gender identity. In these cases, implants are an excellent solution. There are, however, a few threats, both real and perceived, to successful lactation that come along with them and that bear discussion.

There are several factors in the implant procedure (medically referred to as *augmentation mammoplasty*) that might impact how much it will affect lactation. Starting at the beginning of the procedure, there are a few different techniques used for the primary incisions, but meta-analysis research (Cheng *et al.*, 2018) has shown that we have no reason to believe that any of them will specifically affect lactation outcomes.

Implant location is a different matter, however. There are three main options here: subglandular (the implant is in between the glands of the chest tissue and the pectoralis muscle), submuscular (the implant is behind the pectoralis muscle) and dual-plane (the implant is partially under the muscle and partially under the glands). There are some more specific variations your doctor may refer to, but for our purposes these are the big three. There are multiple considerations to discuss with your doctor when determining what is best for you; but of these, submuscular tends to be the least problematic for lactation. This is because of the way pressure is dispersed on the milk ducts and glands. When the implant is pressing directly on them as with a subglandular or dual-plane implant, it can cause atrophy because they are being constantly squashed. That being said, it's important to remember that there are thousands of milk glands and ducts, so even if several are damaged you may still be able to produce a full supply of milk. In a ten-year observational study, approximately 20% of all patients had insufficient milk production regardless of their incision or implant site (Jewell *et al.*, 2019).

Whether the implants contain silicone or saline does not seem to be especially relevant to lactation outcomes or milk quality. There were some studies in the 1990s raising concern about silicone leaking and contaminating milk, which you may have heard about, but those studies have since been redacted due to flaws in the research. Furthermore, infants are far more likely to ingest small amounts of silicone from other environmental sources and most of it will simply be passed out of the body without problems.

Other difficulties, such as damage to nerves during surgery and *capsular contracture* (which is when scar tissue forms around the implant itself), can lead to lactation issues; and while it's important to consider these eventualities in your decision making, they are largely impossible to predict and control for (Erickson-Schroth, 2022).

Reduction
If you're wondering about how top surgery specifically can impact lactation, see my detailed discussion in Chapter 2. However, reduction

procedures are also often done for other reasons, such as simply relieving physical or emotional discomfort that may be associated with having a large chest. When talking about inducing lactation after reduction procedures done for these reasons, the important things to remember are that you will have better lactation outcomes if the NAC remains intact and if a specific effort is made by the doctor to avoid removing glandular tissue and to focus on removing adipose tissue. However, this will likely impact the appearance of your chest after surgery, so you will need to decide for yourself what your priorities are in that regard. Many people choose to postpone reduction procedures until after they give birth for this reason.

Trans men who choose to induce lactation also face the potential difficulty of dysphoria. Since inducing lactation is a voluntary process, why would anyone do it if it makes them dysphoric? Bryna discusses their professional experience:

A lot of the time when I'm working with somebody who is trans masc, I'm working with them because they want to lactate for personal or for kink reasons. And they want to be able to do that safely. And, you know, obviously, not everybody experiences dysphoria, but that's something that's always a consideration because it often does happen and it really depends on their goals, what they're inducing lactation for, and also what their T levels already are. A lot of the time people have been on T for a long time, and so it's really about adjusting the profile to maintain as much T as possible while still allowing lactation to occur. I find that their experiences are really similar to experiences of somebody with PCOS, for example, somebody with really high androgen levels.

People can make milk; it's just about how much milk, and how much inflammation is introduced into the system. Whenever we cause that system to work again we see an increase in inflammation, which sometimes is definitely worth it. We just want to kind of balance that out. I think that that can make a huge difference.

Will I be able to make all the milk my baby needs?

I can't give you a definite "yes" on being able to produce all the milk your baby needs. However, if you have so far read all of Part 2 and don't feel as if you have any conditions which may cause difficulties, you've never had surgery on your nipples, and you're generally healthy, I do feel comfortable giving you a "probably." Even if not all of those things are true, the answer would still be "maybe," and I'd remind you that any amount of your milk is a wonderful gift. Even holding and latching your baby with supplemental milk or holding your baby to your bare chest without latching has physical and emotional benefits for both of you.

What if I begin inducing but have to stop?

The good news here is that no matter what step you get to in the process of inducing lactation, if you ever need to stop or postpone your lactation journey for any reason, there are no permanent physical effects that will impact future lactation. If anything, the knowledge you have acquired about lactation and your body will aid you in the process should you choose to continue or restart later on.

How do I know which pump to get?

As discussed earlier in this chapter, those of you inducing lactation will almost certainly want to get a pump of one kind or another. For this reason, I'm putting all of the information about pumps in one place, although some of it will only apply to those who have given birth.

People tend to think that pumps are 100% necessary for all babies who are exclusively fed human milk, but remember that these are a relatively new invention in the grand scheme. For many people, feeding your baby on demand will be your best bet for a full supply. Regardless of all the advancements in pump technology, there is no pump that is anywhere near as efficient as a baby at removing milk.

Whether you should get a pump or not depends mostly on your lactation goals. The majority of families I work with do opt to buy or rent one, especially if it is covered by insurance, so the option of using it is available to them. You may never use the pump if your baby is getting all of their milk directly from you or if you decide to cease lactation shortly after birth. However, it would be prudent to accept one if it's offered or find a place local to you that rents pumps just in case. Lactation clinics, pharmacies, and clinics which focus on AFAB (assigned female at birth) health are places to inquire about rental pumps. This way, if you change your mind or there's an unforeseen circumstance, such as an illness or infection which requires short-term separation or you have an out-of-town emergency, you won't have to scramble to find one.

If you are planning on having other people bottle feed the baby, you want to have a stash of milk in the freezer for hospital visits (planned, unplanned, or emergencies), or you are planning to return to work or school, then a pump is necessary. So, what kind of pump will you need? There are a few things to consider when picking out a pump, but the good news is that they all work basically the same way: there's a small motor with a piston that creates a vacuum, the suction travels through tubes to the flange, which then stimulates your nipple to express milk. In other words, pumps don't pull milk out, they create suction which activates your glands and ducts to release milk. The milk then gets funneled into a small bottle.

An important note is that the companies which make pumps don't seem to be particularly concerned about inclusive language, so if you're feeling emotionally fragile you may want to steel yourself before browsing online. Below are a few of the main things people talk about when they discuss pumps.

Insurance pump

If you have medical insurance and the insurance company knows you've just had a baby, they'll probably send you a pump or information on getting one. In my experience, over the last few years, insurance companies have become pretty relaxed about people requesting a pump to induce lactation and will just send you one if you ask for it, but you'll need to check with your company to see what their policies and protocols are.

I can't be too specific about the quality of insurance pumps since typical makes and models vary depending on your carrier and may very well be different by the time you're reading this; but I'm fairly comfortable in saying that the pump options they are providing are probably pretty good. Also, you have already paid for the insurance pump.

Borrowed or gifted pumps

If a friend or family member offers you the pump they used when they were lactating, that pump is probably also pretty good. There's definitely something to be said for the warranties and customer support that come with buying a new pump, but if you get offered a free one and it seems to be in working order, take it (as long as the pump is a closed system, meaning that milk only ever touches the replaceable parts). I recommend that you purchase a new pump kit (everything that isn't part of the machine) just to be on the safe side and to avoid cross-contamination or if your nipples are a different size from the previous owner, but it's not strictly necessary if all the parts are sterilized before use. You can buy a sterilizer or special bags for sterilizing parts in a microwave, and most pump makers will have instructions for sterilizing their kits on their website.

Hospital-grade pumps

When you're looking around to buy a pump a term that comes up a lot is *hospital grade*. This term doesn't have a specific meaning, so you'll never find a definitive list of hospital-grade pumps. What it *generally* means is that the pump is good enough to be used in a hospital. Which is to say, it's a closed system safe for multiple people to use without cross-contaminating milk and the motor is good enough that it can go for several hours a day.

Insurance pumps are generally not hospital grade because they don't have to be. If you're the only one using your pump, the motor doesn't have to be great—just good enough for 20-minute pumping sessions a few times a day for a few years at most.

Any of these mechanical pumps are also likely to have a massage or letdown setting which should not be ignored. The purpose is to stimulate your nipple and areola just enough to trigger your letdown reflex so you start expressing some milk before it starts the more intense, rhythmic suction.

Manual pumps

If you want to go the minimalist route, you can also look at a manual or hand pump. It works on the same principle, except instead of a motor and piston there is a lever that you use to create and control the suction. The advantage here is that you have total control. The disadvantage is that you have to do all the work, and you can only pump one side at a time. Some folks like to have a manual pump for use outside the home, in addition to an electric pump for home.

Hand expression

Another route for having total control is hand expression, which I discussed in a previous chapter. This method involves massaging your chest to stimulate milk production, and unlike the other methods there is also a little bit of directly squeezing the milk out. There are special containers you can buy to catch the milk which you hold with one hand while you massage with the other, or you can set up a bowl or cup on a table so you massage with both hands and the milk will drip directly into the vessel.

If you are pumping or hand expressing one side at a time—and you may also find this true when feeding your little one—don't be surprised if your other nipple begins to leak. If you're worried about losing this milk, or you just don't want it getting everywhere, there is a product called a *milk collector* which is designed for just such eventualities.

With any of these pumping options, you can feed the fresh milk to your baby immediately, put it in a bottle to use in the next few days, or put it in a storage bag to freeze for later. No matter which method you use, you'll want to avoid transferring the milk between containers more than is necessary. When you pour milk from one container to another, some fat will always get left behind and even though it isn't much, every calorie counts with little babies.

I think my pump is broken

No, this isn't a question but when you work in a lactation clinic you do hear it a lot. If your pump is having a hard time maintaining suction, but isn't giving you any reason to believe the motor is broken (e.g. an unpleasant noise or burning smell) then the problem almost certainly lies with one of the plastic bits between the machine and the bottle. Before you start looking for a new pump, here are a few things you can check out:

- Make sure nothing has a visible hole or crack.

- Make sure nothing is warped and everything is attached snuggly where it's supposed to be.

- If everything is good, the problem is almost certainly the valves between the flange (the bit that goes on your nipple) and the bottle. There are a few different designs but regardless they are the last piece to ensure a vacuum is being maintained. If the valve does not look like it did when it was new, you're really going to need a new one. You can probably order a set from the company website or get them if you have a local lactation or infant supply store.

Conclusion

For almost everybody, you have every reason to believe that you can lactate. It may not be easy, but there are people who are here for you. Be patient. While it's helpful to talk with people who are on a journey similar to yours, try not to compare yourself too strictly with other parents, especially if their lived experience is markedly different from your own. Each person is so different, it's all but impossible to predict how your journey will go. It may seem as if your life is a repetitive cycle of pumping and not pumping, and it kind of is. But it won't be forever and one day you'll finally get the big payoff of by directly feeding your infant.

As the *Tao Te Ching* says, "a journey of a thousand miles begins with a single step" (Laozi, 2008). In the journey of inducing lactation, learning about the process and starting to think about your plan is the first step, and by making it this far you have already begun. Maybe you're ready to continue now, in which case, congratulations! I encourage you to reach out to a professional or other people in your community who have induced lactation or relactated, get a pump, and just start experimenting with what works for you. Remember, you don't want to overwhelm your body or mind.

CHAPTER 7

An Inducing Lactation Deep Dive

During my interview with Bryna, they spoke extensively about the importance of patients knowing their own bodies and monitoring hormone levels via blood work, particularly for their trans femme patients who are inducing lactation and those who had not previously been using any hormone treatments.

There are a couple of really interesting studies out there that look at this through working with the trans population, particularly trans women but also folks who are trans nonbinary, and gender expansive folks who are assigned male at birth. There's a study out of New Orleans where trans women were inducing lactation with herbal protocols and working almost entirely outside the confines of the medical establishment, for obvious reasons (Glick *et al.*, 2018).

But the most important thing is to find a provider, especially a prescribing provider who can be really supportive, to maximize your chances. That's not to say that people can't and don't do it on their own. Most people are doing it on their own. But knowing what your lab work looks like is a huge help because then you can use whatever method that you're planning on using to increase your estradiol and progesterone level, and know what your peaks and troughs are, how fast your body processes progesterone, which is wildly different across the board. I've seen the lab work of the folks that I work with, and figuring out the timing of your dosing so that you can spend time developing that glandular tissue which people don't often stop and contemplate [is so important]. They often want to go straight to pumping and domperidone while also just beginning the birth control, and that is not always necessary. Domperidone isn't always necessary, because if you have the estradiol level correct for yourself, and you have the cycling and timing down, a lot of the time your pituitary will take over and your prolactin level will increase *endogenously*, on its own.

A lot of people think that they have to follow a protocol that's been established, without understanding exactly what they're doing and why. It's about self-education and it's also important to access the work that others have done. The grassroots calculator Transfeminine Science is amazing for calculating hormones. This is an anonymous, self-contributed dataset that thousands of people have put their levels into. It can calculate, based on your dose and your timing and a couple of other things, what your blood levels will be for a certain hormone. It's really cool because it helps people who don't necessarily have a knowledgeable provider to work with. It helps them to go from not knowing to knowing and using the right dose. They then have that time—I find that it usually takes between three and six months to establish and develop glandular tissue, depending on where somebody is in the hormonal milieu of their transition space. A lot of people transition without using any sort of hormones at all, either through lack of access, lack of resources, or lack of interest. And so, a lot of people are starting from scratch and need to proliferate some mammary tissue to begin—and that can be a huge hurdle.

It's about knowing about your heart and if you have a longer QT pause, an interval between the Q and the T on their electrocardiogram readout. (*Note: simply put, the QT interval is the time between your heart contracting and relaxing each time it pumps.*) And so, when you're looking at that heartbeat, basically there's an interval between the Q

and the T, and what domperidone can do, and for some people definitely does, is increase that interval, and that can be pretty serious.
If someone doesn't already have an extended or elongated interval,
they're unlikely to have that side effect. But I think domperidone
has been oversimplified as being judged as unsafe. And so people
say, "Oh, it's been decided that it's unsafe. It's black boxed because
they don't want us to use it," which is also true, but there's a lot more
that goes into it. There is an actual risk. There's also quite a significant risk of an increase in dysphoria and other perinatal mood and
anxiety disorders. And it's been implicated in exacerbation of even
postpartum psychosis, so all of those things need to be considered.

The other thing that I would say to really increase your success
is to work with a therapist. I make sure that everybody I'm working
with has access to some type of therapist. It doesn't need to be a formal therapist if they can't find someone who's safe, but they need to
find some sort of professional mental health support, either within
mutual aid, within their community, or online. Because the risk of
dysphoria with these changing levels of hormones, even if they're
changing in the direction that is affirming, can still be an issue. For
example, dysphoric milk ejection reflex, which is a different type
of dysphoria, but is still very severe and significant, as well as perinatal mood and anxiety disorders, which you don't have to give
birth or gestate to experience. So it's quite a complicated path to
travel completely alone and there are a lot of pitfalls along the way.
I think that one of the things we do is to find communities all on our
own. Really, we've had to. And the problem with that is within that
community, sometimes we have a bunch of folks, with wonderful
intention, putting information out without understanding the risks
that come alongside it. But it doesn't mean don't do it. It just means
that you need to understand what these risks are and how to do this
as safely as you can.

CHAPTER 8

Case Studies

Inducing lactation case study 1: Coral's story

Coral (she/her) is a parent who induced lactation and was kind enough to find some time to speak with me, even with her new baby. Coral's story is a good example of the limitations of the Newman-Goldfarb Protocol being designed for cis women. Although inducing did not work as well as she had hoped, she was able to collect more milk with hand expression than either of the pumps she tried and continued to latch her child utilizing a supplementer. Following her story are a few pieces of advice she has for other women on inducing lactation.

It's not a great time for trans healthcare. The doctor that I was seeing was not even really a trans doctor, just a doctor that some trans people went to. I had mostly just been going to him to get my hormones and he didn't really have to do anything. It was a pretty uncomplicated thing for him. So when I brought up trying to induce lactation and that I would need to change my hormones, he was just kind of freaked out by it. He basically refused to offer care in that way.

I followed the Newman-Goldfarb Protocol, so I think I started taking domperidone maybe four or five months before my kid was born. It was kind of hard to find a doctor who would work with me, but I finally found one who worked with me to change my hormone regimen. I basically just shifted my hormones and started taking progesterone and increased my estrogen quite a lot. And I did that ramped up for, I think, two months, and then I was on a pretty high dose for a little bit, and then I tapered off the progesterone and way lower estrogen and just kept taking domperidone the whole time. About eight weeks before my baby was born, I started pumping, eight times a day, including in the middle of the night. And then I increased to basically doing between 10 and 12 pumps a day, just before they were born.

It was really hard to pump because I was also working. I'm on parental leave now, but I was trying to fit it into my schedule at work, which was pretty challenging. So it was just hard in all kinds of different ways. I also didn't really react very well to pumping. It didn't really do what the protocol said it was going to do or even what the studies said had happened for other women. It was also just quite discouraging to be doing something so many times a day that wasn't having a lot of effects. I was very rarely making milk that would even hit the bottle when I was pumping. It was more like drops for quite a long time. And that actually never really changed with pumping. I'm not even pumping right now because I found that doing hand expression was way more effective for me. Nowadays when I hand express, on a good day, I probably get a little bit more than an ounce at one time. And the lowest is probably like half an ounce; before I was hand expressing I wasn't getting very much at all.

I've been using the supplemental nursing system. I was giving them some donor milk from a friend, but then we switched to formula. So I've just been doing formula in the supplemental nursing system and that's been working out pretty well for us. I don't actually know how much they're getting from me each time, but it still feels nice and feels as if it's basically facilitating the same thing even though I wish I had enough milk to feed them that way. It just didn't work out like that.

I changed a lot of my first goals: that I wanted to fully feed them just from my body and that we would do that until they were ready to wean. But that's not been the case. I haven't totally reassessed what my goals are. I really enjoy breastfeeding them and I think they like it too, so I'll probably continue to do it for some amount of time and go back to work in a few months. I'll probably do it at least all the time that I'm not working. When I'm back at work, I'll have to assess if I'll just do it a couple times a day or if I'll just stop doing it altogether. I'm not exactly sure.

I feel that one piece of advice would be to talk to someone who has already been through it. It would have been helpful to hear do this, don't do this, talk to this person, if you say this to this person you can get access to domperidone, if you ask these kinds of questions to this kind of doctor, they're probably not going to be helpful—these kinds of things.

I think another thing that is probably relevant for all people who are inducing lactation is to have very low expectations about how the process might go, because it seems as if it really varies for different people. I was very disappointed in the beginning that I made such a small amount of milk.

Also have flexibility. I was trying to follow the protocol in the way that it was set up, and it was confusing to me that the pumping didn't work or didn't seem to make a difference; but the hand expression was really useful. That's probably something that would be hard to tell someone unless you had a really experienced lactation consultant that you were working with. But that was just from me experimenting with different things, not only going off what I was told to do. I think that has been my experience of being a trans person in this world in general. You just need to experiment with different things because what is offered is not necessarily what's right for everyone.

I really wish that there was a different way for trans people to be connected about this kind of stuff, because the whole process has been very challenging. I hope that more resources emerge from this work that you're doing too.

Inducing lactation case study 2: Rebekah's story

Rebekah (she/her) was the first person I had the pleasure of interviewing for this book. As you will see, physically her experience of inducing lactation went as well as could be expected, but there were unforeseen emotional difficulties we hope you can benefit from learning about.

I followed the Newman-Goldfarb Protocol pretty much to a tee. I was on birth control and domperidone for a little over six months and I did start pumping a little early, which I didn't need to. I think I was just excited at the time. I started pumping about ten weeks or so before my daughter was born rather than the six weeks they recommend.

I dropped the birth control and then 24 hours later I started pumping. I think I was pumping every three hours. At the time, I was working as a postpartum doula overnight and I was able to pump at night a couple of times, so I had a pretty full pumping schedule. I pretty much pumped around the clock for the first three-to-four weeks, and when I started having large quantities of milk it was like, okay, I think I'm not going to be so aggressive with the pumping.

The schedule I ended up with for six-to-seven months was pumping every three hours during the day and then once overnight. And slowly I dropped the overnight pump. It was easy to pump overnight when my daughter was a newborn because my wife would feed her and I'd be up changing her and stuff so I just pumped while my wife was feeding her.

I ended up reaching an average of 30 ounces a day within, I don't know, probably five-to-six weeks with the pumping. I have a lot of milk storage. I went through a lot of galactagogue-like supplements and herbs. I found that goat's rue was extremely helpful. I think I was two months into the protocol, I had been on birth control and domperidone for two months and, you know, people say that you're looking to feel fullness in your breasts, or tenderness. I hadn't really felt much and I wasn't concerned at the time, but I was just interested and had read somewhere that goat's rue worked similarly to milk ducts and so I added in goat's rue and within like a week I had very tender breasts, very swollen and enlarged. And so I continued on goat's rue the entire time I was on the first part of the protocol before I started pumping.

Once I started pumping, I did keep the goat's rue and I added in shatavari and moringa [*always check with a medical professional about drug interactions, especially if you are taking multiple herbs*]. I think those were the two main ones I added, and I know I experimented at different times in that initial stage and during pumping, adding in Dairy Fairy and Pumping Queen or something like that from Legendairy supplements [*after this interview, I received a follow-up email clarifying that the supplement from Legendairy was called* Pump Princess]. But I never really stuck with one supplement apart from goat's rue and shatavari because I ended up making so much milk in the long run that I wasn't desperately trying to increase my supply, I was just trying to maintain it.

Before the baby was born I felt very like, okay, I'm checking all the boxes. Everything is going according to plan, so great. I think it's when you add another human into the mix that things go a little less as expected. It was something that I presented to my wife before we even got pregnant and she was like, "Yeah, that sounds cool. I didn't know that was possible. Let's do that."

So she was on board. As I induced, she was continually impressed that so much milk was coming and so fast. She had questions as we got closer, because she was definitely planning on nursing herself. How are we logistically going to handle this? You have enough milk for one baby and I want to make sure I have at least enough milk so we can nurse 50/50? And that was also a question I had at the time. I was in a lot of Facebook group stuff, and I really hadn't found many other co-nursing parents who planned on nursing 50/50 or both of them fully nursing as much as possible. So I was kind of navigating it mostly on my own, trying to figure things out and set us up for success. My plan had been that when our daughter was born, to have my wife nurse the majority of the time for the first week or couple of weeks to one month, to make sure that she established her supply, and I would continue pumping during that time and then just comfort nurse as I was able. That was the plan going in. But it didn't necessarily work out exactly like that.

When my daughter was born, everything went pretty smoothly with my wife breastfeeding. And I did latch my daughter once or twice the day she was born and then at least once a day for that following week. But my wife, I can't remember what day it was— probably day four or five postpartum, when obviously emotions were really high—started having this internal feeling of jealousy when I was nursing. She was having a really hard time watching me nurse.

It wasn't like her at all, so it was really challenging to navigate, especially with high postpartum hormones. And me, really excited to have a baby that I had dreamed of nursing my whole life, but also really wanting to support my wife however possible and make sure I understood that she was going through a lot.

That started our journey of trying to figure out how to co-nurse and, in the end, it didn't really work. My daughter started refusing to latch onto me at around six weeks old so I just pumped until my daughter was about six months old. We had so much milk and no need for all the extra, so I ended up weaning off the pumping.

I think the most challenging part I have found is that almost no one else talks about that jealous feeling. It wasn't a rational feeling. She was totally on board with me nursing through the whole pregnancy. Giving birth, she was on board with the plan. We attribute it to hormones, similar to postpartum depression. Something was just telling her, "I need my baby and I don't want someone else to be nursing her." But it was too complicated when that someone else was your wife. That was the challenge we ran into. We found ways to try to manage it: I would nurse my daughter once a day, in a different room while my wife was sleeping or resting so that it wasn't really on her mind when it was happening. And that worked kind of, but because of the nature of breastfeeding she would most likely have to pump during that time. It was still a reminder that someone else was nursing her baby.

I think it was about two weeks postpartum when we went to our midwife. They were also fully on board with inducing, even though it was new to them. We tried to explain to our midwife what was going on and ask, "Do you have suggestions? Do you attribute this to the hormones or is there something else going on?" And she just had no idea and no answers for us. That was really challenging because she had been the person we had looked to our whole pregnancy for questions, and even she didn't have an answer. I wasn't finding an answer on Facebook groups or even any similar stories that I could relate to. It definitely caused a lot of tension in our marriage in those early days because there were times when my wife, very high up with postpartum hormones, was like, "You just have to quit breastfeeding. I cannot handle that added on with this newborn baby," and I was like, "You don't understand what you're asking me to do. I've worked so hard for this. I can't just stop."

That was really challenging and it was hard not having anyone to relate to or anyone to go to who could understand. Because we have interesting relationships with our families, they're not really on board with our marriage in the first place, so we couldn't go to any of them. They definitely would not understand or be supportive. Even some of my friends who are midwives—I was consulting with them—just said, "You have a really unique struggle and it does sound as if she's having really high hormones or even the baby blues or postpartum depression." When we tried to address that with our midwife, she gave my wife the test that asks ten questions [*this is called the Edinburgh Postnatal Depression Scale and can be used to determine the emotional wellbeing of gestational and non-gestational parents*], trying to identify if she had postpartum depression. From her answers to the questions, she didn't, but it felt as if she was in a depression when we were discussing that issue.

My daughter is a little over two years old now. My wife very much recognizes that it was driven by hormones, "That wasn't really my rational thinking, but I still don't know how I would have done it differently. It was almost like a primal instinct of, like, I need my baby."

We continued with me trying to nurse my daughter once a day for about six weeks, but because my wife always seemed to have a pretty strong let down, my daughter quickly started getting fussy when I was trying to latch her. We suspect it was just because she was used to a really quick flow and she did not like having to work for her milk. So I would have to work really hard to get her to latch and that just furthered the tension. My wife would say, "If we're making her this upset, just let me nurse her." Then one day the baby completely refused, and I never got her to latch again.

I did try. It was challenging, I didn't really want to try much when my wife was around so I tried here and there, in a dark room, when she was sleeping, but none of it really worked. Ultimately, I knew that she was having a really healthy nursing relationship with my wife. She was thriving and they loved nursing, so I just continued to pump.

I ended up donating to a lot of friends in need, which I think was fulfilling after such a long road and it not going the way I had planned. It was nice to be able to donate so much milk to a lot of families.

Inducing lactation case study 3: Taylor's story

Taylor (she/her) had only been taking hormones for a few years when her wife became pregnant and she decided to induce lactation. In addition to the usual stressors, this was also during the height of the Covid-19 lockdown and the George Floyd protests.

The earlier you can start in your partner's pregnancy the better. I think that ultimately what did it, or didn't do it, was that I waited until they were four months pregnant. We just didn't think of it before that really, or I didn't make the decision quickly enough. Also, I had only been on hormones for two years at that point so it was pretty early in my breast development. That probably had an impact too. There wasn't a lot of breast tissue. There was *some*, and more grew. It is quite good for breast development actually.

I was pumping multiple times a day, the recommended amount. Before she was born, my mental health was fine. Honestly, we had a really great pregnancy. And that all went pretty well. We got one of those automatic pumps, and I was using that multiple times a day. It was funny because we drew little eyes and a mouth and taped them to the pump and gave it a little face because that's just a cute little thing. That was before the baby was born. I'd say my mental health started to get worse about three weeks after the baby was born.

My profession is social work, and the term that we use that resonates with me is *role strain*. I've had a hard time adjusting to motherhood because of all the sacrifices it requires, the changes that it requires you to make in your life, the loss of your individuality, your independence and stuff. And, when she was born, it just became very real—there was a big fire in Australia at that time, and there was a lot of chaos going on in the world, so I was like, "What did I bring my child into?" Not that I didn't know that already, but it just became more real. So between that and the role strain, my mental health started to decline and I stopped pumping as regularly as well.

By the time the baby was actually born in May 2020, the Covid-19 pandemic had started. My mental health took a hit during the pandemic, so I probably didn't do as good a job when she was born as I could have. We tried to get it to work, we tried a supplemental nursing system when it didn't take initially, but she didn't really like it, so I gave up after a few tries. I think if my mental health had been a bit better I probably would have kept trying because the suction can obviously help the milk come.

I think, by that point, my doctor had already moved, so, against my partner's advice, I stopped the domperidone without weaning off it well enough and that really increased my negative mental health symptoms. I can't say for sure, but it seemed to. So I was not okay for a little while, because of not being able to make it work, because of the hormonal change, and other societal factors and whatnot.

I had been an activist in the past, so when the George Floyd protests started happening, I felt a sense of loss from not being able to participate in a way that I would have wanted. I did help remotely organize a street medic group for some friends of ours. I would run the Discord and stuff, so I was pretty involved with that for a little while, but then eventually my mental health got bad enough that I wasn't really able to continue. I basically engineered myself out of a job at that point. I recruited people who could do the work that I had been doing and changed my focus to completely at home because I didn't have the bandwidth to do anything else. That's pretty much all of that story.

PART 3

GENERAL LACTATION INFORMATION

CHAPTER 9

How the Body Makes Milk

Like just about everything else the human body does, lactation begins in the brain. People are often surprised to learn that pretty much everybody has the various glands and organs necessary for lactation. The hormones that cause lactation (prolactin and oxytocin) are made in the pituitary gland, so nearly everyone can make them. Although there are certain disorders of the pituitary gland that may impact a person's ability to produce milk, they are incredibly rare. The pituitary gland also helps to regulate estrogen, another key part of the lactation process.

The majority of the time, when a person lactates it is because they recently gave birth or are currently pregnant. That is what this chapter focuses on (lactating without becoming pregnant is discussed extensively in Part 2). Although there is some variation, the generally agreed on terms for the different stages of milk production that lactation professionals use are: *lactogenesis 1*, *lactogenesis 2*, and *galactopoiesis* (which means *milk producing*). This third stage is also referred to as *lactogenesis 3, autocrine control, or lactogenesis 2, second phase.*

Lactogenesis 1

In the same way that everyone is born with nipples, everyone is also born with the glands, ducts, and alveoli which make and distribute milk. They just don't really do much until a person becomes pregnant, and at certain times during their menstrual cycle. When pregnancy starts, massive amounts of estrogen and prolactin in the body start kicking things into gear, initiating lactogenesis 1. This stage is also called *secretory differentiation* because it's when all the cells lining the inside of the alveoli (the epithelial cells) differentiate into cells that make milk (Wambach & Spencer, 2019). Within just a few weeks after a person becomes pregnant, estrogen and progesterone begin activating the milk ducts that have so far been dormant. Prolactin then begins converting the epithelial cells into *lactocytes*, which are cells that make and store milk. At around 12–13 weeks after gestation, they start making colostrum, which can be thought of as a nutrient-dense precursor to milk.

Why don't pregnant people start lactating during pregnancy? See, this is the tricky bit, because while progesterone and estrogen activate the ducts and glands, they actually suppress milk production, and are sometimes called *lactation antagonists* (Deakin University, 2019). While some hormones are activating cells and making milk, other hormones are specifically keeping that milk inside the body until the baby is born.

Lactogenesis 2

When the baby and placenta are delivered, progesterone quickly drops all the way back to baseline. Now the prolactin can commence making colostrum (and later milk) in larger quantities. People often describe the first three days after birth as when their "milk comes in." Lactation professionals call this *lactogenesis 2*. Within a few days, the estrogen levels fall down to baseline, and the prolactin levels fluctuate but stay well above baseline unless or until milk stops being removed (Wambach & Spencer, 2019).

When milk is removed, either by feeding or pumping, the pituitary gland increases prolactin and starts producing oxytocin.

The prolactin increases the amount of milk being produced, and the oxytocin makes the milk cells contract and eject the milk through the nipples. This happens in waves, often with a tingling sensation called *letdown* or the *milk ejection reflex* (MER), which can happen multiple times per feeding session.

In the hours between feeding or pumping sessions, prolactin is still relatively high, so the *feedback inhibitor of lactation* (FIL), which is not a hormone but a whey protein that is part of the milk and exists only in these cells, slows down milk production to avoid too much from being produced. As the name indicates, it inhibits the feedback loop responsible for the supply and demand system that is forming (Deakin University, 2019).

It's important to know that each side of the chest has its own feedback loop, so it's ideal to remove milk as evenly as possible in order to maintain an even supply. A common trick is to keep a hair tie around a wrist on the side the baby just latched on to.

Galactopoiesis

Usually within about two weeks after delivery, the body acclimates to regulating these hormones in new ways, and the person begins to develop a schedule or routine of milk removal. A supply and demand system begins to form. As mentioned earlier, this stage is also referred to as *lactogenesis 3, autocrine control, or lactogenesis 2, second phase*. Until now, milk production was based on the hormones made and regulated by the body's endocrine system, so it was under endocrine control. Now it has more to do with cells telling each other to make more milk, so it's said to be under autocrine control. The new prolactin baseline decreases, and milk is predominantly made during the surges of milk removal. FIL levels become lower as the body regulates prolactin more and with some regularity.

Involution

Presumably, at some point, the person will want to stop producing milk. This is clinically referred to as *involution*. Because milk production is based on supply and demand, simply slowing and eventually stopping milk removal will reduce milk-producing prolactin levels and allow the FIL to begin inhibiting again. At this time, progesterone and estrogen levels increase again (Deakin University, 2019). If any pain or discomfort is experienced at this time, it is best to contact an IBCLC or other lactation professional.

CHAPTER 10

Questions about Your Nipples and Chest

The rest of Part 3 will be delivered in a Q&A format, covering a variety of extremely common questions and those that are less common but very important. The first set of questions are about anatomy, mainly having to do with the nipple, areola, and chest tissue itself. These will be followed by questions about milk and milk production, questions about pumping and bottle feeding, and finally questions about babies and getting milk into them.

Does the size of my chest/nipples matter (if I haven't had surgery)?

The size of your chest and nipples is not as important as you might think in terms of milk production or milk removal. Chest size mostly has to do with adipose tissue, whereas milk production and storage has more to do with the glands and ducts, which, until recently, were microscopic. You have no cause for concern if you are small chested.

The same is true of nipple size. I have never heard of anyone having nipples too small to latch their baby; more common is having nipples too large to comfortably fit in your baby's mouth, which is rare but does happen. This can be problematic and you may have to pump or hand express more than you had initially planned, but it is usually self-correcting given the quick rate at which newborns learn, grow, and adapt to their environment. Regardless, the size of your nipples won't have a significant impact on how much milk your baby is receiving. If you're concerned about your nipples being too small, think about it in this way: maybe the number of milk duct openings you have is on the low end of average (average is often considered 15–20 but some studies indicate the range may go to as low as 4–18) and your baby is working harder than others to get milk. Your baby doesn't know that. As far as they're concerned this is the way it is for everyone. As long as they're cool with it, no worries.

If you're reading this and not pregnant but thinking of becoming pregnant and you're concerned about your chest size, remember that the chest, nipples, and areolae will almost certainly grow quite a bit during pregnancy.

There is one particular condition called *insufficient glandular tissue* (IGT), which is a condition of the endocrine system that can impact the ability to lactate. Onset can be at birth, puberty, or pregnancy, but it's fairly easy for a professional to diagnose due to a characteristic look; the chest tissue is widely spaced and can be tubular, with bulbous nipples. Folks with this diagnosis would benefit from seeing a lactation consultant to discuss their feeding goals and needs, but, as revealed in my interview with Kristin-Cole, this is not a deal-breaker:

> I have IGT and of course I didn't know. So I had a starving baby who was under birth weight at six weeks. It was incredibly traumatic for everyone. And I had six different IBCLCs telling me that nothing was wrong. Actually, five told me nothing was wrong, then finally the sixth one did a weighted feed. So no one had done a weighted feed on my under-birth-weight baby until number six, and number six found that he only transferred a quarter of an ounce in 45 minutes. So yeah, I had to figure everything out by myself pretty much and I ended up being on domperidone, which was helpful.

At one point, I think I was taking like 30 pills a day of different stuff. And I used a supplemental nursing system and donor milk. He ended up nursing until he was almost six years old.

I have extra nipples, will milk come out of them?

Maybe. If you have supernumerary nipples, they may be developed enough to have milk come out of them during lactation depending on their size and where they are on your body (they almost always occur on an area called the *milk line*, which runs between the armpit and groin). If they are more fully developed, you may have *polymastia*. This often occurs in the armpit, but can also be on the ribs or closer to the groin and can occur on just one side or both. There's no way to know if milk will come out of them, or if they will swell with milk but not have an outlet until lactation begins. If they do lactate, you can get them to stop producing milk without affecting your total production by applying cold packs. I would definitely do this with the guidance of a lactation professional.

My nipples are innies. Is that going to be a problem?

Whether or not inverted nipples pose complications to lactation depends on how inverted they are but it's never a full on dealbreaker. Clinically speaking, there are four types of nipple inversion:

- *Minimal retraction.* Your nipples look pretty flat, but pop up pretty easily when you're cold or aroused.

- *Moderate to severe retraction.* The nipple looks flat and you need to physically pinch the areola to get the nipple to evert.

- *Simple inversion.* Your nipple really looks as if it's going inward, but you can still get it to come out if you apply pressure (sometimes called the *pinch test*).

- *Complete inversion.* The nipple looks similar to simple inversion, but no amount of manipulation will cause eversion. It simply inverts further. This is extremely rare. Any nipple inversion is found in only 1.7–3% of the population and, of those, only 4% are complete inversion. If you are lactating with complete inversion, a lactation professional can help you with a tool called a *nipple shield*, which is placed over the nipple and gives the infant something to latch onto when feeding (Wambach & Spencer, 2019).

What about piercings and tattoos?

Having pierced nipples will not impact your ability to produce or express milk. In fact, you may end up expressing milk faster out of a nipple that has extra holes in it. That being said, there are a few things to consider regarding nipple piercings:

- If you previously had a piercing and it has now healed over, the resulting scar tissue can cause blockages in the milk ducts. Due to the prevalence of nipple piercing in our culture, there is a lot of reported data that has been collected by various journals. The consensus seems to be that *some* people have problems but *most* do not. Whether or not you will have problems seems to be impossible to determine ahead of time except that the more scar tissue you have, the more likely it is to cause a blockage (Armstrong *et al.*, 2006; Garbin *et al.*, 2009).

- If you have a nipple piercing at the time when you have a baby, take the piercing out before you feed the baby. Some people just take their piercings out for a few months while their baby will spend a lot of time latched; some are content to take them out and put them back in several times a day, but never latch your baby while you have a piercing in. It can fall out and be swallowed by the baby which can be a choking hazard or seriously damage their still-developing digestive organs.

- If your nipple piercing is relatively new (remember that it takes 12–18 months for a nipple piercing to fully heal) I would recommend just taking it out and deciding if you want to get repierced after the baby has weaned.

You may have heard that you shouldn't get tattoos while you're making milk, but the people who say that often leave the reasons why up to the imagination. I have talked to people who were under the impression that ink would make its way into their milk. Rest assured, this cannot happen, but there is one very good reason to hold off until the baby has weaned; tattoos (and piercings) are, in a very real sense, wounds which can become infected. While the chance of infection probably doesn't change if you're making milk, it does create one more thing for you and your body to take care of.

Why do my nipples leak sometimes, even though I've never even been pregnant?

The word for spontaneously making milk is *galactorrhea*, and while it is most common among people who have been pregnant or previously lactated, there are a few reasons it might occur in someone who has not. If your nipples only leak when you're aroused or they are being stimulated sexually or by clothing, then it is referred to as *idiopathic galactorrhea*, which means that it's just the way your body responds to the prolactin hormone that is always present. While it doesn't necessarily indicate cause for concern, you should let your doctor know just so it's on your medical record. Unfortunately, there is nothing you can do to prevent it from happening besides avoiding the behaviors that cause leaking.

A sudden onset of galactorrhea may also be something to discuss with your doctor. This can be caused by certain medications, such as birth control pills, antidepressants, antipsychotics, sedatives, and high blood pressure drugs. However, it could also be a symptom of a hormonal imbalance or other problem with your chest tissue, thyroid, pituitary gland, kidneys, or spinal cord (Wambach & Spencer, 2019).

Is it weird if one side makes more?

You might find it surprising if one side gradually starts making a lot more than the other, or if they've always kind of been that way; but I can assure you that, in the general scheme of things, this is both common and normal. The cause is probably related to your anatomy; maybe the side producing less happens to have fewer milk glands, perhaps a fall or car accident several years ago caused internal damage you didn't know about until now; there are myriad possibilities. One side producing slightly more can also become something of a self-fulfilling prophecy. You or the baby may favor that side, so more milk is being removed from it, so it continually produces more milk. If you want to counteract the effect, simply make a concerted effort to start with the side producing less milk and favor that side until you even out.

If one side starts making more all of a sudden, I would recommend making a note of it but not worrying too much unless it continues for a week or more. If one side decreases all of a sudden and you're also experiencing pain or discomfort, consider seeing a lactation specialist.

What is that whitehead on my areola?

It's not quite a whitehead but it is similar in that it's a clog in your areolar glands. It has an absolutely amazing name: *bleb*. The areolar glands secrete an oil which helps your baby locate the nipple but they can get clogged, much like a pore. It may also be a clog in the milk duct, but very close to the surface. Either way, they often come out naturally when you're removing milk or feeding your baby.

Should it hurt when I pump or the baby is latched? When should I see a lactation consultant?

Before I get into the two different parts of the question, I think it's important to clarify what I mean by "hurt" or "in pain" versus "discomfort." If this is your first time lactating, you've got a bunch of glands and ducts doing things they've never done before. Many of them are going to begin swelling. It's going to be uncomfortable, it will probably ache, perhaps more than you anticipated. Discomfort may be in new sensations or uncomfortable tugging that subsides pretty quickly as your body gets used to the new routine of feeding. You probably don't need to worry about this. Pain, on the other hand, will be persistent, may increase over time, and indicates a latch or chest issue that needs to be addressed.

In the case of discomfort, a slight adjustment of your body or the baby's body may be in order, or perhaps you need to relatch. When you're first starting out with bodyfeeding, discomfort is both normal and common so is not necessarily a cause for concern; but whether or not it's "okay" is really up to you. Try the things you usually use for body aches and cramps and, if it doesn't get better, go and see a professional.

If this is your first time chestfeeding or pumping, you might be surprised by how much attention is being paid to your nipples, and it's going to take a bit of getting used to—emotionally, mentally, and physically.

If you find you can't get used to it, or if you're experiencing direct, localized pain anywhere in your chest region, I recommend contacting an IBCLC for a consultation. Even in more complicated situations that might involve other professionals (like tongue or lip ties or mastitis), IBCLCs can teach you strategies for feeding through these challenges and preventing future pain. Pain directly on the surface of or within the nipple or areola should be reported to a lactation professional quickly, as it could be various types of bacterial or fungal infections or a *vasospasm*, which is caused by an interruption in blood flow to the area. All of these are usually easily treated once you know what you're dealing with.

If you're experiencing pain while pumping, but not when the baby is latched, you almost certainly need to make an adjustment with your flange size or pump setting. As you pump, your nipple shouldn't be rubbing against the inside of the flange, as that will lead to chafing. If you're not sure what flange size to use, most pump companies have sizing guides on their website. When setting the pump suction, a good rule of thumb is to turn the pump suction up until it feels just a bit too intense, and then turn it down one notch. Remember that pumps aren't made to pull milk out, just to stimulate you to express milk into the bottle (Berens *et al.*, 2016).

What about cracking/chafing?

Nipple chafe is not just for runners. If latching or pumping feels scratchy, burns, or is consistently uncomfortable, you need to make some sort of adjustment before it gets worse. Chafing is not a self-correcting problem, and you don't need to "toughen up." If you're pumping, this might just be a question of adjusting your settings (speed and suction), getting a new flange size, or using some coconut oil as a lubricant. For chestfeeding, adjusting the latch or position is your best first step. If you can't fix it on your own, seek support from a lactation professional who can offer you some advanced tips your parent friends may not be privy to and help assess whether there's something going on with your baby's mouth.

Tongue ties are relatively common, lip ties are less so, but each of these restrict movement of the baby's tongue or lip and can lead to nipple chafing, as well as inefficient feeding. These challenges are sometimes called *tethered oral tissues* (TOTS) or, clinically, *ankyloglossia*. The good news is that the procedures to correct ties are fairly quick and common practice through a pediatric dentist (LeFort *et al.*, 2021).

If my chest feels soft, does that mean there's no milk?

Even if your chest never really feels as if it's full of milk, it's important to remember that the chest didn't evolve to store milk so much as make milk. Much of the milk is made as it's being removed, so as long as your baby is eating well, seems happy, and is gaining weight appropriately, don't worry if your chest doesn't feel like you expected it to.

If I'm producing milk, should I be worried about weird lumps?

If you notice a lump in your chest tissue or armpit it's probably lactation related and benign but you still might want to see a lactation consultant about it, especially if you're experiencing other symptoms such as heat, pain, or discoloration of your skin, which could indicate an infection. Either way, you should keep latching your baby or pumping. Even if you do have an infection or growth of some kind, your milk will still be fine for the baby and removing the milk may help clear out a clogged duct. With that in mind, my first course of action would be to see if you can break up the mass by gently massaging it with your fingertips or vibrating it with a vibrator or electric toothbrush. You may also be able to clear a duct by latching the baby, having their chin line up with where the clog is (if physically possible). Some people are able to recruit their partners for this task, if the baby can't line up with the timing or positioning. If the mass can't be broken up or removed, definitely make an appointment with an IBCLC and they can either identify it or refer you to a doctor who can make a diagnosis.

I say this to offer you some peace of mind; depending on your medical history there are about a dozen things it could be besides a tumor. Even if it is a growth and you've never had surgery or any trauma to the area, it could just be a random cyst or abscess, which are more common during lactation (Mitchell *et al.*, 2019).

CHAPTER 11

Questions about Milk and Milk Production

Most of the questions I receive as a lactation professional come from parents concerned about the quality or amount of their milk. It's very reasonable to worry if any pre-existing conditions or treatments for conditions will have an impact, especially if feeding your child your milk is extremely important to you. I've done my best to collect as much information as possible on illnesses, medications, and lifestyle factors and how they affect milk safety; if anything is not covered, please consult a medical professional.

Will my medication affect my milk?

I will always recommend that people err on the side of following the advice of medical professionals, but, generally speaking, there are some medications that affect how much milk you produce, and a few will have an effect on the quality of your milk; however, even taking these is not necessarily a dealbreaker for providing your milk to your child. Some of the more common ones include certain selective serotonin reuptake inhibitors (SSRIs), such as Celexa and Prozac, as well as pseudoephedrine, which can hinder lactation in the short term for the same reason it dries your sinuses. Pseudoephedrine does not generally have long-term effects if you maintain regular milk removal. Any time you are given radiation therapy or radioactive isotopes it is recommended that you dispose of your expressed milk until the radiation has cleared from your body (Sriraman, Melvin, & Meltzer-Brody, 2015).

Even if you received anesthetics during labor or delivery, if your baby is healthy, you can latch them as soon as you are ready and feel able. Some medications need as many as six-to-twelve hours to stop affecting you, but, during that time, you can pump and then mix that milk with milk you express later to further dilute the small amount of medicine that may be present. If you need anesthetics later but while you are still making milk, let the doctor know that you're feeding a child and request that you not receive opioids. Although small doses will not affect your milk too much if this is not possible, it's best to err on the side of caution (Reece-Stremtan *et al.*, 2017).

Will drugs/alcohol affect my milk?

I want to be really clear here: this information is just regarding specific instances of use while you are a lactating parent. This information does not pertain to pregnancy or long-term drug addiction. This is to answer questions like, "If I drink some beers or eat a gummy, is my milk safe?" Also—and I cannot stress this enough—do not personally try to feed your baby if you are impaired or might pass out. If it is at all possible, ask someone else to help. Let someone else take care of your baby when you're high or drunk. Beyond that, drug or alcohol use is rarely a dealbreaker for giving a baby your milk, but let's talk about some specifics.

Alcohol

Drinking alcohol while pregnant is generally discouraged pretty much across the board and people tend to behave as though drinking while lactating is the same. We know from lab tests that the amount of alcohol present in a person's milk is almost exactly the same as their blood alcohol level (Reece-Stremtan & Marinelli, 2015). So if you've had two drinks in an hour and your blood alcohol level is about 0.04% that means the same amount of alcohol is in your milk, but remember that it's going to keep breaking down. Even if your baby needs to be fed immediately, that's actually fine. It's an incredibly small amount of alcohol (approximately equal to half a teaspoon of alcohol in a gallon of water) and studies show that the only immediate drawback is that your baby may eat slightly less, but then they'll just eat more later.

The main problem with feeding your baby while you've been drinking is that you're impaired regarding motor skills and decision making. Put simply, you're more likely to drop the baby if you're drunk. Accidents happen, but outside that, don't try to handle a baby while you're drunk or high.

Nicotine

Regardless of whether nicotine gets into your system via smoking, vape, gum, or a patch, it's known to constrict blood vessels and therefore decreases the rate of milk ejection and milk volume. Since most people who use nicotine do so regularly, it's unclear how long this effect lasts. Actual exposure to second-hand smoke is of course bad for everyone but especially infants and toddlers. It goes without saying, but I'm going to say it anyway, never hold a baby while you have a lit cigarette.

Several studies indicate that there is a correlation between shorter duration of lactation and smoking, but it's worth noting that these people may have been given the instruction that they need to quit one or the other and nicotine is a powerfully addictive chemical they may have been dependent on for decades before giving birth (Reece-Stremtan *et al.*, 2017). While quitting smoking is always ideal, if the choice is between making milk for your baby as a smoker and not making milk for your baby, keep making milk for your baby.

Caffeine

Caffeine transfers pretty readily into milk and then into the baby, who is fairly bad at metabolizing it so it tends to stick around. It's unknown whether there are long-term effects, but it's well documented that caffeine will keep babies awake. If tea or coffee is necessary for you to be a functioning human, you might consider cutting back as much as you can and having it only in the morning so that it will be out of your system well before the baby goes to sleep at night (Wambach & Spencer, 2019).

Marijuana

Outside the previously discussed reasons to not smoke around infants and children, there are also concerns regarding whether it's safe to ingest other forms of marijuana while you are making milk for your baby.

While clinicians are almost always going to discourage use, it's important to specifically talk about why. Even with occasional use, THC (tetrahydrocannabinol, the active ingredient in marijuana) stays in your system for days, which makes research difficult since researchers can't know how much a person is using specifically. This also means that waiting for it to clear out of your system, as you might do for alcohol or caffeine, isn't a practical option. Most people who use marijuana while lactating also used it while pregnant, which also complicates research.

All of that being said, we know that the THC in cannabis causes changes in the cannabinoid system in the brain (which is, in fact, how the cannabinoid system was named) and that every part of an infant's brain is extremely underdeveloped compared to an adult's. Therefore, even small amounts or occasional usage may have long-term detrimental effects on an infant, although research is not specifically clear on the subject, and if it is a choice between occasionally using marijuana while providing milk for your baby or not providing milk for your baby, definitely keep making milk. Again, just wait until you're sober to hold the baby (Reece-Stremtan & Mar-inelli, 2015).

Other drugs

If you take any other drugs which have not been prescribed to you, the most important consideration is the substance's half-life, which is how quickly it breaks down in your system.

For most pharmaceuticals, the half-life is both easy to find and predictable (a quick online search reveals the half-life for ketamine is 2.5–3 hours, for Xanax 11–13 hours).

For substances which are naturally occurring or made illegally, a half-life is less predictable. For example, when people talk about mushrooms, they're talking about more than 75 different species grown in different conditions so there is really no way of knowing how much psilocybin (the psychoactive compound) is in any given

Table 11.1

Drug name	Half-life	Half-life x5	Half-life x7	Risk level
Cocaine/crack	1 hour	5 hours	7 hours	Very high risk (APILAM recommends 24 hours)
Ecstasy	15 hours	75 hours (3 days + 3 hours)	105 hours (4 days + 9 hours)	High risk
Mushrooms	3 hours	15 hours	21 hours	Unclear
Morphine	3 hours	15 hours	21 hours	Low risk
Heroin	2 hours	10 hours	14 hours	Very high risk
Methampheta-mine	17 hours	85 hours (3 days + 13 hours)	119 hours (4 days + 23 hours	High risk
PCP	51 hours (2 days + 3 hours)	255 hours (10 days + 15 hours)	357 hours (14 days + 21 hours)	Very high risk
LSD	21 hours	105 hours (4 days + 9 hours)	147 hours (6 days + 3 hours)	Very high risk
Ketamine	3.1 hours	15.5 hours	21.7 hours	Low risk

batch (Aronson, 2016). When one takes LSD or ecstasy, it's impossible to know the exact potency or any other substances it's been cut with. Furthermore, for some drugs, there is little or no research on how much of it will transfer to a person's milk. The Association for the Promotion of and Scientific and Cultural Research into Breastfeeding (APILAM) currently maintains a database of drugs and supplements, showing how they interact with milk.

Table 11.1 shows common recreational drugs and how long they recommend you wait before giving milk to your baby (APILAM, 2002). This number is based on the rate the substances break down (half-life); at 5x the half-life a substance is 96.9% gone and at 7x it is practically non-existent. Also included is the overall risk level rated by that organization. If you're uncomfortable disposing of your milk, you can always freeze it and use it later to make soap or lotion for you or your baby.

Will illness affect my milk?

Generally speaking, no. For most common illnesses, your milk will actually be more beneficial to the baby because you'll be providing them with antibodies. For certain severe illnesses (e.g. tuberculosis and chickenpox), your doctor may recommend that you wear a mask when you're feeding or pump your milk and have someone else feed the baby (Meek & Noble, 2022). In some cases, it may be prudent to pump and dispose of your milk due to the medication you're given. As of this writing, the only illnesses for which there is a blanket recommendation against infant feeding are: ebola, a bacterial infection called *brucellosis*, and certain types of T-cell lymphoma (Kamali *et al.*, 2016; Meek & Noble, 2022). If possible, you should seek aid with childcare if you have any symptoms which impair your decisions, such as very high fever. Also, avoid latching your baby in any context where you would avoid skin-to-skin contact, such as if you have a herpes sore, poison ivy, or similar rash on your nipple or areola.

Regarding infant illness, the only one which entirely forbids human milk is a metabolic condition called *galactosemia*. This is a very rare condition some people are born with that makes them unable to digest the galactose sugars found in human milk (Meek & Noble, 2022).

What about HIV?

The advances that have been made in the detection, treatment, and prevention of HIV and AIDS are truly remarkable; however, it is still a disease of particular concern to all queer communities.

While the evidence is consistent, global agencies vary in their recommendations about how to proceed if you are HIV positive and want to provide milk for your infant. Bear in mind that the guidance all starts with something to the effect of, "If you are on antiretroviral treatment *and* the virus is undetectable..."

In *Updates on HIV and Infant Feeding*, published by the World Health Organization and United Nations Children's Fund, it is recommended that parents lactate "for at least 12 months and may continue breastfeeding for up to 24 months or beyond (similar to the general population) while being fully supported for ART [*antiretroviral treatment*] adherence" (2016 p.19).

In *Recommendations for the Use of Antiretroviral Drugs During Pregnancy and Interventions to Reduce Perinatal HIV Transmission in the United States*, the United States Department of Health and Human Services recommends the following:

Achieving and maintaining viral suppression through antiretroviral therapy (ART) during pregnancy and postpartum decreases breastfeeding transmission risk to less than 1%, but not zero.

Replacement feeding with formula or banked pasteurized donor human milk is recommended to eliminate the risk of HIV transmission through breastfeeding when people with HIV are not on ART and/or do not have a suppressed viral load during pregnancy (at a minimum throughout the third trimester), as well as at delivery.

Individuals with HIV who are on ART with a sustained undetectable viral load and who choose to breastfeed should be supported in this decision.

Individuals with HIV who choose to formula feed should be supported in this decision. Providers should ask about potential barriers to formula feeding and explore ways to address them.

Engaging Child Protective Services or similar agencies is not an appropriate response to the infant feeding choices of an individual with HIV. (Panel on Treatment of HIV During Pregnancy and Prevention of Perinatal Transmission, 2023 p.E-11)

In the UK, the National Health Service has a framework called "The Safer Triangle," which indicates that as long as the parent has an undetectable viral load *and* no cuts, lesions, or infections on their nipple *and* neither the parent nor baby has diarrhea or nausea, the baby can be fed directly from the parent exclusively for up to six months with only a 0.3% chance of infection (National Health Service, 2023).

Will exercising affect my milk?

If exercise is important to you, especially from a mental health/self-care perspective, you can rest easy knowing that from a lactation perspective, you can resume your routine whenever it feels good to do so without significant impact to your milk production. I would recommend pumping or feeding your baby just before you work out if possible. It will certainly be more comfortable and also you may find your child reacting to taking your milk immediately after you work out, since minor changes to your water and sodium levels may make the taste slightly different. They should acclimate pretty quickly, however. You should definitely take into account the water and calories you burn while exercising, in addition to your already increased need because you're lactating. You might find that you're eating and drinking pretty much constantly.

Will my diet affect my milk?

The short answer here is "no," your diet won't affect your milk production in any meaningful way. The milk your body makes will be what your child needs nutritionally regardless of what you're eating. You may notice minor differences in the color, aroma, or taste of your milk if you've been eating foods that are particularly strong in those regards, but as long as you're getting all the recommended vitamins and minerals, which can be done by taking a multivitamin, you don't need to worry about all of your food being made from scratch, being nutrient dense, or certified organic.

You're already making all of the food for your new little one directly with your own body, so if feeding yourself is causing undue stress, just eat what you like and have time for. I will stress, however, that staying hydrated will go a long way to making sure you're producing enough milk and feeling good while doing it.

Will drinking cow's milk help me make more milk?

This comes up periodically, and while it certainly doesn't hinder milk production, there's no indication that drinking milk from cows or any other animal increases the amount of milk your body can make. It is worth noting, however, that if you are going to drink milk, make sure it's pasteurized. I mentioned a bacterial infection called *brucellosis* being a reason to stop chestfeeding and the main way that people who do not work with animals acquire that bacteria is through raw dairy.

Does sleep training affect my milk?

Will sleep training affect the quality of your milk? No. Will it affect the amount of milk you produce? Probably. I say this because often, a parent's goal when they initiate sleep training is to be able to have six-to-eight hours of uninterrupted sleep every night. In theory, this is fine and there's no reason to believe it will have any long-term negative health impact on your baby, but if you also want to maintain a full milk supply, then you can't really go that long without removing any milk.

In my opinion, if you're willing to wake up in the middle of the night to pump you might as well take the opportunity to feed your baby instead, but you may have individual considerations I'm not aware of. With a little bit of luck and practice you'll be able to feed your baby without waking them all the way up and this will help them sleep later in the morning.

It may seem as if it's taking forever, but remember that everyone sleeps through the night eventually.

Will having a cesarean section affect my milk?

For the sake of keeping this simple, let's say that there are two main ways of delivering a baby, via the birth canal or cesarean section (there are variations in each of these, but that's not relevant right now). Regardless of how your baby comes out, the hormonal shifts triggering lactogenesis 2 are going to occur, so in that sense the method of delivery is irrelevant to milk production. However, what will often affect lactation is what happens immediately after delivery, in a time often referred to as the *golden hour*.

About 25% of hospitals in the US and 43% of maternity services in the UK are accredited by an organization called the Baby-Friendly Hospital Initiative (BFHI). There are currently 20,000 facilities in the world designated Baby-Friendly. The reason I bring this up is that at these facilities, the staff are required to facilitate immediate skin-to-skin contact and latching unless it's medically prohibited for some reason. They are also required to educate new parents on infant hunger cues and make sure they have access to lactation support and care. These are hugely beneficial in helping parents achieve their lactation goals (Wright, 2019). If you're not delivering at a hospital or your hospital is not accredited by the BFHI, I would recommend letting the staff and your support team know about your priorities to make sure you are starting off in a way that furthers your goals.

If you're not sure what your goals are or how to accomplish them, attending a childbirth education class or speaking with a lactation consultant ahead of time will definitely be helpful. Your insurance provider may have specific classes they cover, or there may be local groups that can help you find something. There are also a lot of online options, both live and pre-recorded. Unless specifically advertised, childbirth classes and lactation classes can't generally be assumed to be inclusive of gender-diverse parents, so vetting them ahead is always prudent.

One of the most important things you can do to encourage a chestfeeding relationship is skin-to-skin contact immediately after birth. Literally as soon as possible, put that little baby on your chest and let them find your nipple to get their first latch. The oxytocin burst will also help your uterus contract back to its usual size (Wilson-Clay & Hoover, 2017).

If you're under anesthetic or have just had surgery (e.g. a cesarean section), it's important to note that this is not a dealbreaker for skin-to-skin time. In fact, taking this time to begin bonding with your baby may be a good way to keep yourself distracted while the doctors complete the surgery. Depending on the anesthetic used, you may need help from your support team, but that's what they're there for. No anesthetics will have lasting effects on the baby, or are contraindicated for lactation as long as the parent feels well and clear headed (Reece-Stremtan *et al.*, 2017).

Another consideration for parents who had to have surgery of any kind, but especially abdominal surgery, is that usual positioning methods for latching your baby may not work for you. You may want to look into lying-down positions, or modify the regular positions to suit your own comfort.

If, for some reason, you are unable to be with your baby, but you still want to make sure they can have your colostrum, you can always hand express it and collect it in a small syringe to feed to them later. The technique will be the same as with prenatal hand expression, which I discuss in the next question.

How can I produce more milk?

For people trying to increase their milk supply, there are two main methods. As we have discussed, milk is made on a supply and demand basis, so increasing the amount of milk being removed should lead to more milk being produced. If you're already pumping regularly, adding one or two pumps during the day can often increase your overall daily output. For parents who are combination feeding (that is, a combination of formula and milk), try to pump every time the baby has a bottle, if it's practical. This will help your body acclimate to milk being removed more times throughout the day. If you are exclusively bodyfeeding, pumping for five-to-ten minutes after the baby has finished should have a similar effect. It's okay if little to no milk is being collected initially. When you're pumping, doing things to intentionally increase your oxytocin levels may also help. Some ideas include having a picture of your baby or other loved ones around your pumping area, having something that smells like your baby nearby, or lighting a soothing scented candle. Playing music or sounds that you find soothing or bring you joy may also help stimulate letdown. One time during a group session when I mentioned oxytocin, an individual who had given birth as a surrogate about six months earlier asked me if they should masturbate while pumping to produce more milk. Choosing my words carefully I responded, "I'm not going to tell you to masturbate while you pump. But if you choose to, it probably wouldn't hurt your milk production." Do with that information what you will.

Another piece of advice comes from AJ, who reminds us that sometimes we can lose focus on what the most important details are:

> "Watch the baby, not the clock." That's an oldie but a goodie. And that doesn't just mean don't look at the time, it means so much more. "Oh, the baby has lost four ounces," Okay, but were you worried before we knew about those four ounces? Is everything else going really well? Is baby growing, is baby crying, is baby sleeping, how are baby's bowel movements, and is everything else okay? The clock detail is supporting evidence, but it's not the most important factor about lactation and whether it is going well and whether it is successful.

If you're generally having a hard time producing milk, make sure that you're getting all your vitamins and minerals and are staying well hydrated. The quality of your milk won't change, but your body will produce more milk if it has all the nutrients to maintain itself. I recommend lactating people to continue taking any prenatal vitamins you were already taking. If you're vegan or vegetarian, you might want to look into taking an iron supplement and B vitamins, which pretty much everybody could stand to have more of. The reason most things considered to be milk-producing foods or *galactogogues* work is because they are either high in B vitamins or are calorie-dense foods like cookies. I've provided two tables in Chapter 5 of the most common foods and herbs said to aid in milk production, with a bit of information on each. It is worth noting that a review published in the *Journal of Human Lactation* included research done on galactagogues and found none that had sufficient evidence to begin recommending them clinically (Mortel & Mehta, 2013).

Another technique is to give your chest a little pre-feeding warm up. Using a fist or the palm of your hand, rub or pat your chest starting at the clavicle or armpit and moving in towards the nipple. Do this a few times, rotating around your entire chest area. The idea is to start activating the milk ducts and generally get the party started.

Don't some people make too much milk?

Yes, although what counts as "too much" will change as your baby gets bigger and needs more calories. There isn't usually a physiologic cause for *hyperlactation* or oversupply, it often happens when a parent is doing all the things to make sure they have enough milk and just overdoes it. The good thing about this is that it's pretty easily managed by storing the excess milk for later and slowing down milk removal. If you're doing any pumping you can just cut out one or two sessions a day. If the baby is getting all your milk directly, it's a little bit trickier. First of all, ease up on the galactagogues if you're taking any.

If none of this applies to you but you're still producing a lot more milk than your baby needs, I would recommend seeing a professional. They may recommend a technique called *block feeding*, where you only feed from one side at three-hour intervals during the day, instead of both sides during a feeding session. So from 9am to 12 noon feed left, from 12 noon to 3pm right, from 3pm to 6pm left, and so on. Night feedings can still be on both sides, and it's usually recommended you only do this for a day or two at a time. If you experience discomfort or don't see any improvement, they may recommend some herbs or over-the-counter medicines that hinder lactation (e.g. peppermint, sage, or pseudoephedrine) or refer you to a doctor to see if it is a hormonal imbalance (Johnson *et al.*, 2020).

What are the other uses for milk?

If you do have a lot of extra milk, infant care and lactation professionals (and enthusiasts) love to espouse the many uses for human milk besides just feeding babies. As AJ says:

> I'm a real strong believer in there's no such thing as unusable milk. You can use it for loads of different things other than feeding directly to the baby. You know, one of the first things I say to clients who are pumping and storing milk is get a takeout container or an old bottle or whatever for your milk that can't be drunk. Because you can save that for baths or, you know, making nappy ointment or whatever it might be.

People will variously claim that it can be used topically for almost any skin ailment you or your baby may have, ear infections, and even as a treatment for cancer! As you may expect, some of these claims can be considered overblown at best. However, some are fairly accurate, or research has shown that milk works about as well as an over-the-counter ointment and you already have it on hand, so to speak. Let's go through a few of the claims you're more likely to encounter.

- *Ear infection.* This is not exactly true, but I think the reason it's so widely believed is really more of a miscommunication than anything. Ear infections usually occur beyond the eardrum, so drops of milk in the ear won't do much. This is why they require a visit to a medical professional to remedy. However, feeding your child your milk has been shown to decrease their likelihood of getting ear, nose, throat, and sinus infections. This is most likely due to the antibodies you're sharing with your baby (Li *et al.*, 2014).

- *Skin problems.* In various studies, applying human milk topically to skin irritations, such as diaper rash, acne, eczema, and cradle cap, has been shown to be about as effective as using a 1% hydrocortisone cream.

- *Nipple wounds.* In controlled studies, human milk did not work any better than lanolin (the conventional recommendation) in curing nipple trauma. However, as I previously mentioned, it's worth a shot because you do have it right there.

- *Umbilical cord care.* In multiple studies, umbilical cord separation happened faster when human milk was applied then ethanol, chlorhexidine, or leaving the area to dry.

- *Eye problems.* Human milk has been found to promote faster healing when used topically on infants with conjunctivitis (pink eye) or minor corneal wounds.

- *Cancer treatment.* Human milk is used in certain cancer treatments, after it's been highly altered. One of the compounds in human milk, alpha-lactalbumin-oleic acid, can be modified in a laboratory specifically so that it causes cancer cells to break down. This new compound is called *human alpha-lactalbumin* made lethal to tumor cells (HAMLET) and successfully shrank bladder and colon cancer cells in mice.

Even though human milk sometimes works and sometimes does not, research also indicates that it's almost always worth trying a topical application of human milk if you have some available.

> [Human milk] involves no risk of allergy, contains antibodies, ep-idermal growth factor (EGF), and erythropoietin, which may pro-mote the growth and repair of skin cells. Human milk is a source of commensal bacteria that can play an anti-infectious, immuno-modulatory role. Their possible function in the acceleration of con-ditions for skin biofilm formation can open new perspectives for the prevention and treatment of skin and wound healing diseases (Witkowska-Zimny *et al.*, 2019).

Given milk's usage as a topical remedy, it probably won't surprise you to learn that there are also people who make soaps and lotions out of extra milk. Recipes are pretty easy to find, but writing about *all* of the different things you can do with milk would be a whole other book.

Is it okay if my milk is any color other than white?

In general, yes, it's normal for milk to be different colors. Milk comes in a wide variety of colors, and for the most part exclusively chest-feeding parents don't know what color their milk is at any given time. The only time to be particularly concerned is if your milk is bright neon pink as that indicates a specific bacterium, *Serratia marcescens*, which can cause various infections in the parent or child. In this case, don't panic but call your doctor, who may prescribe you an antibiotic.

If your milk is any of the following colors, this is probably why:

- *Clear:* Early milk is often clear because it has more water and protein and less fat than the milk you'll produce later.

If you're pumping, you may even notice changes in the milk color from the beginning of the pumping session to the end of it, when the milk becomes fattier.

- *Redish (dull pink to brown):* If you've just started lactating and your milk is red, orange, dull pink, or brownish, this may be due to the unfortunately named *rusty-pipe syndrome*. This is caused by small amounts of blood in the ducts being swept up and expressed out with the milk. While the thought of it can be off-putting, it's harmless to your baby and usually resolves itself within a few days.

- *Yellow:* When people think of milk, they expect it to be white, which makes perfect sense since cow's milk is white. But fat is naturally yellow in color (think butter) and human milk has about 25% more fat in it than cow's milk (depending on a number of factors). So a creamy yellowish color may be more common than pure white most of the time.

- *Green:* Green milk almost always has to do with the food and supplements the lactating parent is eating. If you're taking herbal supplements or eating lots of leafy greens to get your iron and folic acid up, some of that chlorophyll may have ended up in your milk.

- *Blue or gray:* Gray or grayish milk is perfectly normal and indicates that your milk has more protein in it than usual. Again, the nutrient content of your milk changes throughout the day, so just because it's not your typical color during one pump or feeding, doesn't mean it will stay this way. If your milk is actually blue, it probably has something to do with a food or food dye you recently had a lot of (Wilson-Clay & Hoover, 2017).

- *Black or dark brown.* A certain antibiotic called *minocycline* has been reported to cause a very dark brown or almost black discoloration in milk. The exact cause of the discoloration is not known, and some doctors will prescribe a different medication because of it, but there is no specific contraindication for lactation if you only need a single round of the antibiotics (Hunt *et al.*, 1996).

CHAPTER 12

Questions about Feeding the Baby

Sometimes difficulties in feeding have less to do with making milk, and more to do with actually getting the milk into the baby. Often, these difficulties occur suddenly: one day everything is fine and the next your baby is ravenous or refuses to eat. Generally speaking, neither of these is a problem short term, but knowing what's likely to be going on will help put your mind at ease.

Is it safe to feed my baby in bed?

This question comes up a lot. I think it's important to acknowledge that at some point, you're going to be sorely tempted to take your baby into the bed and feed them there. It's going to be a time when you're already incredibly tired and not thinking clearly about safety. With this in mind, let's consider now what steps you can take in order to safely feed your baby in bed in the middle of the night. Rather than reinvent the wheel, I'm going to defer to the guidance offered by La Leche League International and what they refer to as the Safe Sleep Seven. I edited the original points for the sake of inclusivity, but the spirit is the same.

You are:

- a nonsmoker
- sober and unimpaired
- a lactating parent

and *your baby* is:

- healthy and full-term
- on their back
- lightly dressed

and *you both* are:

- on a safe surface.

If all of these are true, they recommend that you can safely feed your baby on the aforementioned safe surface. This means a bed (not a couch or chair) that doesn't have heavy quilts or comforters, extra pillows or toys, and has no cords or pets. Make sure it's not too far off the floor and have something soft for your baby to land on if they do fall. Make sure the bed is away from the wall and there's no crevice or crack they can get stuck in, falling is better than getting trapped. Make sure there's nothing sharp on the bed or ground, in case they do fall (Wiessinger *et al.*, 2014).

How can I get the baby to latch better?

I think every book ever written on lactation addresses this question, and it's one of the few where the answer is pretty standard across sources. I'm going to assume here that all of the information I'm about to give you is brand new, so if you're one of the readers who has heard this before, please bear with me. When most people say latch better, what they mean is a deeper latch—in other words, getting more of your chest into the baby's mouth. It's surprising how much tissue will fit in there for a good latch.

Let's start by thinking about it in terms of trying to fit something into your own mouth; for example, imagine taking a large bite of a sandwich. First, you take the sandwich in both hands and squash it down so it will fit better. Next, you aim it so you can get the maximum amount of sandwich into your mouth. This part of the metaphor is actually more of a negotiation between aiming the sandwich (your chest) and the mouth (your baby's mouth). It sounds inelegant, but lactation sometimes is. I feel as if it goes without saying (but I'm saying it anyway): this is going to take some practice.

Now we're on step three, open wide. Luckily, there is a trick for getting babies to open wide. Tilt their head back like you do when you're drinking a glass of water and then just give them a little boop on their top lip with your nipple. Most babies will reflexively open their mouth when you do this. You can try it with your finger, bottle, or pacifier if you want, so you know the exact spot on your little one. When you put the sandwich (your chest) into the mouth (baby's mouth), aim your nipple at the roof of their mouth, and, as my mentor used to say, "Shove with love." Throughout this process, make sure you're sitting as comfortably as possible and *bring the baby to you* as opposed to leaning forward to bring your chest to the baby. If you're having trouble with this maneuver, this is another thing that a lactation consultant can help you with.

How do I know the baby is eating enough?

One of the potential downsides to exclusively bodyfeeding is that it's impossible to know *exactly* how much the baby is getting. Sometimes exact numbers can be comforting, but they can also create unnecessary and unrealistic expectations. New parents may be tempted to get a scale to weigh the baby each time they eat, but I have found that unless specific monitoring is medically indicated, it can often exacerbate the anxiety that led you to acquire a scale in the first place. As long as your baby is having wet and dirty diapers throughout the day, seems satisfied after feeding (as in, no more hunger cues—see below), and is growing as expected, you can rest assured that they are getting enough to eat.

A newborn's stomach is very small (about five milliliters, or the size of a teaspoon) but grows rapidly so by day four they might be at a quarter of a cup. If it feels as if you're feeding them all the time, it may be because you actually are! Trust your baby that they will let you know when they're hungry, and they will trust you to give them food and comfort whenever they need it (Wambach & Spencer, 2019).

How do I know when the baby is hungry as opposed to sleepy, grumpy, or in pain?

One of the coolest things about babies, to me, is that, regardless of culture, they tend to have the same ways of letting adults know what they need. If your baby is twisting their head as if they're looking for something, opening their mouth and/or sticking their tongue out (often called *rooting*), or putting their fingers in their mouth, it's time to eat! If these don't work, then the baby might start fussing and squeaking a bit before moving on to crying. If possible, feed the baby at the first hunger cues. They'll latch easier and eat better if they aren't too stressed.

Here are a few tips for how to determine if your baby is communicating something other than hunger, the two most important being tiredness or pain. Babies tend to look tired in the same ways that the rest of us do: a blank expression, droopy eyelids, yawning, and eye rubbing. They do have a few other cues that mean sleepiness is approaching, including pulling on their ears and patting their head (sometimes quite hard!). There are several reasons babies pull their ears, and if they do it a lot it may indicate a health concern, but between the ages of about four and twelve months, ears are just another fun thing to play with and doing so is a form of self-soothing until naptime. Sleepy babies will also either bat their head with their hand (once they develop the motor skills to do so) or repeatedly bonk their head on whatever surface they happen to be on. I've seen some babies who do it quite vigorously, and this can be pretty jarring for parents. As long as they don't seem to be otherwise distressed or uncomfortable and are in a safe place with a soft surface, I recommend letting them figure out how to make themselves comfortable. If you're feeling distressed by this, breathing and focusing on your own nervous system can be supportive to your baby and the overall environment. Helping your baby soothe by rocking, patting, or snuggling can help if they're having a hard time falling asleep, but if they are no longer being swaddled and you try to restrain them while they're soothing, they could end up getting hurt. Again, if it's distressing for you I recommend focusing on your breath as you and your baby navigate this moment together.

If your baby is crying hard and with tears, check to see if there is anything that might be causing pain. The usual culprit, in my experience, is their sharp little fingernails; they may have accidentally scratched themselves. Additionally, check to see if there is a hair or thread wrapped around anything which could be cutting off circulation (fingers, toes, and especially if your baby has a penis); this is sometimes referred to as a *hair tourniquet*. Otherwise, they might just have some particularly uncomfortable gas, in which case a little burping or a tummy massage may give some relief. If they stop crying when you pick them up, they were probably not in physical pain.

This seems like a good time to address the term *colic*, which is used a lot but is often not clearly defined. A fairly standard measure for when a baby is colicky is the rule of three, which is that an otherwise healthy baby cries for more than three hours per day, three days a week, and over the span of three weeks. Sometimes folks assume that their baby needs to be crying non-stop before they seek support, and they try to power through long bouts of crying. However, this doesn't need to be the case; please reach out to your support team for help! We are here for you!

How much time at the chest is too much?

Some people worry that the baby is "using their nipple like a pacifier." I understand why this might be psychologically disturbing or annoying, but *non-nutritive sucking* is perfectly normal behavior for an infant. This is why thumb sucking is common (even in utero) and pacifiers, well, pacify. If your chest feels softer and less full of milk but your baby is still suckling, they are probably just wrapping up their feed. Often, babies won't stay latched for very long if milk is no longer forthcoming. They expect food to come from the nipple, so once that stops occurring, they unlatch and will find something else to explore. However, as long as you and your baby are both happy there is no downside to letting them stay latched as long as they desire.

Is it true that sometimes they just stop eating for no reason?

Sometimes it seems like babies only have two modes: Everything is Great, and Everything is Terrible. At these times, minor changes can make everything go from Great to Terrible. If chestfeeding was going smoothly and then all of a sudden they won't latch, consider if something is different that might be making your baby confused, distracted, or otherwise annoyed. Common culprits are changes to fragrances, such as a new deodorant or lotion, a variation to the usual chestfeeding setup, like new furniture or blanket, or a change to the routine. If you live in an area with daylight-saving time, that can be the problem. Or physical changes, such as ovulation, a change in your diet or medications, or a minor illness in either you or the baby. As long as your baby is getting milk somehow you shouldn't need to contact a doctor; the key to getting through these trying times is just patience at your end. Keep your baby at your chest as much as you can, especially when you're giving them a bottle so they still associate that location and position with safety, comfort, and love. If you start to leak a little while you're giving them a bottle, go ahead and offer the nipple, but don't force the issue. You can also try to use distraction to your advantage. If you start walking around while you feed them, they may have to make more of an effort to focus on you as opposed to when there is just one little distraction and their attention will be easily pulled.

And sometimes they want to eat constantly?

Also true. Babies are wild. You just fed your baby 20 or 30 minutes ago, and they're back to doing hunger cues? Okay, maybe they had a burp or just thought they were done but they weren't. That's fine, they're little and learning how their body works. But what if they do it three or four times in a row? And consistently? Is this just life now? Thankfully, the answer is probably "no." In fact, this phenomenon is common enough to have a name—we call it *cluster feeding*. Most likely, your baby is having a growth spurt and simply needs more calories than usual. It takes a ton of energy to turn milk into more baby, especially if the growth is in their brain, which is about 60% fat (Eliot, 2010). Cluster feeding doesn't usually go on for more than a few days before they learn to re-regulate their eating patterns, so take heart and perhaps you can help them by just letting them linger at your chest for a little while after they initially look finished. This will give them a chance to reconsider so you won't have to start the whole process over again if they decide a few minutes later that they are still hungry after all. If this does go on for a week or more, you might consider calling an IBCLC to assess if something else is the matter.

If you're feeling touched out or as if you could use some time to yourself and there are other caregivers available, maybe you can help the baby learn that skin-to-skin time with them can also be emotionally rewarding.

Also, just because your baby spits up, it doesn't mean they're eating too much. If your baby is getting milk directly from you, they almost certainly are never overeating. Their stomachs are just getting used to milk and how to keep food in. Keeping your baby vertical for 10–15 minutes after feeding can help prevent spit ups, when some of the milk is settled and there is less sloshing around in their stomach.

What can I do if I'm getting bored?

It's amazing what people can get used to and how quickly what seemed magical can become mundane. If you're starting to feel as if all you're doing is feeding your child and cleaning up after feeding your child, remember that with a little practice you can do a great many things while you have a baby latched, even if you do only have one free hand. Here are a few possibilities:

- *Reading a book.* I'm told the trick here is to either get a small paperback you can hold in one hand, an e-book reader, or a great big hardback that will hold itself open. I have a family member who got through the first five *Game of Thrones* books over the course of feeding her sons. Still waiting on that sixth one.

- *Drawing/coloring.*

- *Journaling.* In a few years, you might be surprised to reread what you wrote while your child was feeding.

- *Doing crosswords or Sudoku.*

- *Meditating, but not if you're likely to fall asleep.*

- *Listening to music or a podcast.* Focus on the music you like, not what you think will benefit the baby. Now's the time to get them hooked on your favorite bands.

- *Knitting or crocheting.* I have had friends who do this, which gives me the willies, but they swear they've never poked the baby.

Decide what's important to you and experiment. Where there's a will, there's a way!

CHAPTER 13

Letting Go

Sometimes, despite our very best efforts and intentions, things are not meant to be and there is nothing we can do about it. In the following chapter, we discuss the various options when latching your baby or even producing milk may not be possible. But first, I want to turn the floor over to Victoria, who shares her story of how she came to let go of her plans and is better for it.

I ended up having a really complex birth. Well, it was not complex for most of it, but I had a really rough ten minutes right there at the end. My daughter has cerebral palsy as a result of an injury during her birth. So learning the motor plan of how to eat was actually a tremendous hurdle for her. Because neuroplasticity is so broad, we just don't know when tiny babies are born what their outcomes will be. At the time, we didn't know what her learning abilities in terms of motor planning and stuff were going to be, so now I really understand that her ability to bottle feed was a miracle all its own and was very much a triumph of her motor planning.

I was really attached to the idea that I was going to breastfeed her and that was going to mean something and that was going to, like, save us from this really hard situation we were in. That was going to be the health outcome that was going to change things. That was going to be the reparative experience. I have incredible colleagues, I was at a really phenomenal birth place with really, really skilled lactation consultants, and that was just not going to be on the cards for us. Practitioners whom I love and trust, who are absolute experts in the field and have 40 years under their belt were saying, "This is the most complex case I've ever seen."

And so my journey ended up not being about any of that but being about letting go and accepting what is and loving what is and moving into bottle feeding. But I still was so focused on what I was perceiving as the medical benefits of breast milk that I was white knuckling exclusive pumping in a way that was for me extremely unhealthy and was making my perinatal mood disorder significantly worse. I have pretty significant bodily injury from the birth and that was making it all that much worse.

And so now on reflection, I wish that my future self had been able to come to me and be like, "No, you're actually okay. You could just let this go. This is not going to save anyone and you could just let this go."

And so that is very much part of what my book is, starting from this place of complete failure that we have a culture that prioritizes one kind of eating. No matter how we talk about it, that's just true. And so to be able to say, you know, "I already flunked out of that and so now you are also free to feed your baby, however works for you."

I'm going to be the person I needed and say to you, "You get to do this however you want."

CHAPTER 14

Questions about Pumping and Bottle Feeding

If you're interested in learning about the mechanics of pumps and deciding which is right for you, see Chapter 5 where I discuss that more thoroughly. These questions are more about the experience of pumping and the differences in milk and formula for bottle-feeding parents.

Will my baby get confused if I switch between bottles and chestfeeding?

New parents hear a lot about *nipple confusion*, which is the idea that if a baby takes milk from a bottle, they might not want to latch on to you anymore. First things first: there is no reason to believe that this will definitely happen. Certainly, problems may occur and you should believe the stories your friends tell you about the time it happened to them, but remember that people don't talk about something when everything goes well. For most people who do combination feeding, switching between bottles and latching is a non-event and there is nothing to comment on. However, for those times when it doesn't go as smoothly as all that, remember that human nipples and baby bottles work differently. Bottles don't have the milk ejection reflex, so babies have to suck or squeeze the milk out more actively. They also don't have a letdown, so the milk comes at a more consistent rate and is the same from the beginning of the feed to the end. (Wambach and Spencer, 2019)

Given these differences, your baby may certainly develop a preference for one or the other, and you may need to emotionally prepare yourself for the preference being the bottle. A lot depends on why you're combination feeding. If it's because of a medical condition or difficulty with your anatomy, it may be beneficial for your baby to prefer bottles. If it's more of a timing situation and the baby needs to be able to take a bottle when you aren't available but you'd still like to latch your baby when you are available, then you might want to practice *paced bottle feeding*.

There are a few techniques, but generally speaking this is when you give the baby the bottle at a slight angle so the milk doesn't flow as fast and after they've eaten a bit you adjust the bottle so the milk stops. If the baby is still hungry and keeps trying to eat, you let the baby have some more milk and continue on like this until the baby stops trying to get more milk. This method takes a little longer, but that's kind of the point. The baby is not just instantly getting a lot of milk, so it's more like when they are getting milk from you (Facelli, 2023).

If you're not necessarily wanting to bottle feed the baby, but are having a hard time producing enough milk and need to supplement with formula, you can also utilize a supplemental feeding device, which I discuss in Chapter 3.

If the baby needed to be exclusively bottle fed for a few days and now seems reluctant to latch on as they used to, patience may be the key word. You may need to work with your baby to learn new or different positions or just give your baby time to get used to being at your chest again. Sometimes, if the baby is getting hungry and frustrated, giving them a bottle for a little while, then switching to your nipple when they are feeling more calm will do the trick.

How long will expressed milk be good for?

A fairly standard suggestion that's easy to remember is 4-4-4: milk is good for four hours on a counter, four days in a refrigerator, and four months in a regular freezer. Once a baby starts a bottle, they should finish it within a few hours. If you need to keep milk longer than four months, it should be stored in a deep freezer. Of course, milk is a living tissue and there are multiple variables affecting how long your milk will last. If you're ever in doubt, just treat it like any other milk.

What's a normal amount of milk to produce during a pumping session?

First things first: there are so many little factors that affect how much milk you produce in a single session that fixating on a specific amount or aiming for some generic "normal" can be counterproductive. Worrying about how much milk you're producing during a pumping session can actually make you produce less milk due to the stress hormones. When you're pumping, think about what is normal for you as an individual and focus on the amount of milk you *are* making, not the amount of milk you *aren't* making.

If you are exclusively pumping and worried about the amount of milk you're making, keep track of how many ounces you pump *per day*. If you're bodyfeeding and pumping, there's no telling how much you can expect to pump, and it just becomes a question of how much is typical for you. As long as you don't have any drastic day-to-day changes in volume, and the baby seems satisfied after eating, assume everything is going great!

What's this about donor milk? Is that a thing? Is it safe?

Donor milk is definitely a thing, and can be very safe if you take some precautions. There is an organization called the Human Milk Banking Association of North America (HMBANA, usually pronounced "him-bana"), which collects donations from all over the continent, prepares the milk through mixing and pasteurization, and supplies it to neonatal intensive care units. This example is the absolute safest option, but HMBANA very rarely has excess milk to sell to the general public. There are similar organizations throughout the world; whichever one is local to you may have more to offer. There are also milk banking companies which are just as safe but exclusively sell milk for use outside the hospital. This can be cost prohibitive and inaccessible, however; as of this writing, they charge in the region of $5.00 per ounce, which can add up to $100.00 per day pretty quickly.

The other option is to buy milk from an independent seller. Human milk can be found pretty easily online, but buying and selling is legally questionable depending on where you live. There is also no quality control if you go down this route. You don't know when the milk was expressed or how it's been stored. Anecdotally, people have been known to cut the milk they sell with water (which is dangerous for the baby) or other types of milk (which could create medical complications and you're not getting what you paid for).

An ideal situation for donor milk would be connecting with a family member, friend, or trusted acquaintance who has excess milk they would be able to share with or sell to you. You may ask about medications they are taking, as well as how they pump and store the milk to ensure you feel comfortable. Talking about money in this situation can be awkward, but I encourage folks to remember that producing milk is both a physical and emotional labor and has financial costs associated with it.

Is there really a difference between formula and my milk?

These days, people are often surprised to learn that when companies first started producing a standardized formula the infant mortality rate dropped almost everywhere it was introduced. Before formula, recipes for infant food were mostly bread or cooked grain that had been mashed up and mixed with unpasteurized cow's milk, water, and sugar or honey (Weaver, 2021). You don't have to be a professional to see a few red flags here. Store-bought formula is markedly better than making it at home; however, if you are physically and emotionally able to make your own milk that will almost always be of greater benefit to your child than any formula. If you are not, be thankful to live in a time period when so many people are so invested in making the best substitute they possibly can. Which is not to say that formula does not have problems.

The major problem with formula is that the uniformity it strives to maintain as its main selling point is also the reason it will never be perfect. Once parents find a formula that works well, people don't usually switch brands or types until the baby's needs change. In my experience, most babies who are formula fed only have a few different kinds in their first year of life. And again, knowing that two pots of the same brand contain exactly the same product is what you want in something like infant formula. Human milk, on the other hand, is constantly changing throughout the day and even from the beginning of a feeding session to the end. Throughout a feed, the milk slowly increases in fat content, resulting in what is often referred to as *foremilk* and *hindmilk*. Milk pumped during the day has more cortisol, which is often considered a stress hormone but has the benefit of helping babies stay alert; milk pumped at night has more melatonin, which helps babies sleep (Moyo *et al.*, 2021). These differences are not so great that they are something you should worry about unless your child is having difficulty sleeping or you drink a lot of coffee in the morning. If you're sick, even if you're asymptomatic, in many cases your milk will contain antibodies your child can ingest to prevent them from contracting the same illness.

Millions of years of mammalian evolution really have made it the ideal food for our young.

Unfortunately, we live in a world where it may not be easy for people who cannot make their own milk to readily and safely source milk from other people. For most of us, gone are the days of multigenerational households or friends both emotionally and geographically close enough that they could feed your baby when you are unable. Wet nursing still exists but is not as prevalent as it once was, and you're putting a tremendous amount of trust in someone who you may not know very well. Likewise, donor milk exists, but is often prohibitively expensive or comes from someone impossible to verify. If you do have a trusted friend or family member who is lactating at the same time you need milk and is able and willing to share with you, they are truly a blessing.

The problems that most people seem to have with infant formula are actually problems with formula companies. There is definitely a history of shady business practices, to the point that the World Health Organization has made rules about who is and is not allowed to do business with them, called *The International Code of Marketing of Breast-milk Substitutes* (or the WHO Code) (Weaver, 2021). In many places this is not legally binding, just a code of conduct. In infant care and birthwork, being able to say that you are "WHO Code compliant" is important. Unfortunately, this has led to a great many lactation professionals simply writing off formula as a reasonable option while ignoring other important considerations, as Victoria notes:

> I think it's unethical for IBCLCs to not be really competent in understanding the diversity of families, which includes queer people and the many ways that we feed our babies.
>
> If someone's had top surgery, that probably saved their life and allowed them to have a baby. So we should be affirming formula

as a really awesome, gender-affirming choice for that person just in the same way that inducing lactation can be the same thing on another side.

We're comparing this hypothetical ideal—breast milk as a substance and formula as a substance—which is almost like saying, "Well, if your body produced its own estrogen" then we could compare naturally occurring, cis woman estrogen to a trans woman's estrogen and that's how we decided the risk benefit, but that doesn't work because their risk benefits are different. So if someone doesn't have either the emotional or physical capacity to make milk, instead of *comparing* the two substances, we should be looking at which option leads to their greater wellbeing, and how successful the people are going to be as parents, how they are going to navigate making complex medical choices, and how they are affirming their own experience of identity. This might be gender, it might be work, it might be psychological, it might be that they're disabled and need more rest, or need more sleep. It might be that they have a physicality that doesn't make milk.

It's worth remembering as well that while exact figures are not available, the people at Nestlé, Danone, Reckitt Benckiser, and others are spending millions, or even billions, of dollars in research and development to make sure that infant formula is as good as it can possibly be for your baby. As cookbook author and television host Ina Garten says, "If you can't make your own, store bought is fine."

Can I mix formula and milk?

This is a pretty straightforward question, but sometimes it gets misinterpreted so I want to be very clear. If you're producing milk but still need to use formula to make sure the baby gets enough calories, you can absolutely put prepared formula and milk in the same bottle. However, *do not mix the formula powder with milk instead of water*. It's very important to be clear on this because the result will be too nutrient dense and your baby can end up dehydrated, which can be very bad for humans of such tiny size.

Will formula make my baby sleep better?

Generally, when people ask this question, they're using the word better to mean *more*. So the answer depends on whether the baby is sleeping poorly or just not as much as you want. Depending on your baby's age, there is a range of how much sleep they typically need and how many hours they will typically be awake for, but since all babies are individuals it varies widely. It is true, however, that for the first few months a baby will almost exclusively be either eating or sleeping, with very little in between. If your baby is older than a few months and consistently waking at night, my first recommendation is always to assess their nap schedule, such as it is. They may benefit from having a daytime nap cut out, or if they're prone to falling asleep on walks, they may be getting more sleep during the day than you realize. As previously discussed, parental caffeine intake may play a role in an infant's sleep patterns.

I would also ask whether they are eating well before you put them down for the night. If your baby typically falls asleep while latched, they may be falling asleep before they're really full so they wake up hungry sooner than expected. You might try latching them at the start of your going-to-bed routine, and then again nearer to the end or last thing before you put them in the crib. If your baby has a good nap schedule and eats well right before you put them down but they still consistently wake up hungry after just a few hours, then it does seem like feeding is the answer. Nobody wants to be up in the middle of the night, so if there are multiple parents, discuss who will be in charge of feeding at night. If it's a non-lactating

LACTATION FOR THE REST OF US

parent going in with a bottle, I recommend giving the baby pumped milk instead of formula, if you have any available. But the answer to the question isn't that formula will make them sleep better, so much as more food will, whether it is milk or formula.

Pro-tip: Some studies show that the milk you make at night has more melatonin in it, which helps people sleep better, and daytime milk has more cortisol, which makes you more alert. Marking milk pumped in the evening and daytime might help you to get your baby to sleep better. There are no studies showing exactly how well this works, so I wouldn't recommend being more specific than that, as new parents definitely have enough to worry about. If you find this information isn't helping much and is adding stress, feel free to stop.

CHAPTER 15

Closing Words of Wisdom from Those Who Have Come Before

In writing this book, I wanted to create a space where members of the community could speak about their lactation experience regardless of whether they are lactation professionals or how they had their child. Most of these are words of advice or encouragement but some regard medical interventions. I feel it's important to include these here, but also to remind the reader that they are anonymous personal anecdotes, not clinical data.

- Get really good at asking your community for help. And get really comfortable with the idea of accepting it because we build community by receiving help not giving help. And for many of us, one of the tremendous gifts of being queer is queer family.

- You get to define success. Even some nursing, with or without milk, generates closeness. Even some milk, with or without nursing, is healthful.

- Even though it's a lot of hard work, you can do it, and it's well worth it!

- Have patience and accept what your body cannot do.

- This is going to be difficult. Don't be afraid to keep re-evaluating if it's not working for you.

- Your mental health is important. If chestfeeding is causing you to feel bad mentally, there are other options.

- Do what works for you, and, if you can, take some time to figure out what it is you really want. People have a lot of opinions, but making space for your needs and wants can help determine what you make work; try to block out the other noise. I am glad I took the time to figure out what I really wanted because it has been just right for me and my baby!

- There's too much to write here. But mostly remember that lots of the information is woman-focused so be ready for the endless mama/she/her everywhere.

- You don't have to produce milk to comfort nurse, bond, or show your baby to suckle. You also can produce just drops and it can still benefit your baby! A supplemental nursing system has a big learning curve but can provide a really accomplished feeling once you get it down.

- Find a lactation professional who is part of the community, or at the very least has a proven track record of allyship.

- Listen to your feelings if resources, classes, or any education isn't sitting right with you. You are right to want to be seen and included in the pregnancy/birthing/lactation space and beyond.

- Never stop if confronted with challenges when trying to prepare for and achieve your goal of playing an active role in breastfeeding your children. It's not easy, and many times, when seeking assistance with my desire to serve this role, to have this connection with my future children, I ended up being put on treatment regimens designed with only cis women in mind. I also get a lot of comments about me being male and being able to assist in other ways. So, just don't stop seeking what you need to achieve this goal of being a lactating parent.

- Lactating is hard, hang in there!

- The resources overwhelmingly assume that you are a cis woman! It's important not to compare your experience to cis women's experience if you do not have that experience because it will likely end up making you feel very bad. There are a handful of studies about trans people lactating (I'm a trans woman and I have read about two other trans women lactating) and talking to other trans people who have induced lactation would be extremely useful.

- Do what you have in your heart to do and don't worry about the opinions of others. Or, try not to!

A Brief Overview of Cis Male Lactation

I spend a lot of this book talking about lactation concerns specific to the trans masculine community; however, since my goal is to cover "the rest of us," I feel like it's also important for me to also acknowledge the community of cis men who have lactated or are interested in lactating.

I'm hardly the first person to write about cis male lactation, but when I started researching the subject, I didn't find myself down a rabbit hole so much as on a circular racetrack of a dozen or so articles and book chapters that all cross-reference each other. Therefore, I'm writing this as an overview of the available information and perhaps to offer some new ideas. These writings always seem to tackle one of two questions: can any cis man lactate, and why might they want to?

One of the most cited resources is an article from *Medical Aspects of Human Sexuality* (Greenblatt, 1972), which opens with several historic references:

The Bishop of Cork (1738) observed a 22-year-old soldier from whose swollen breasts 2 ounces of milk could be expressed in 24 hours. Bernhard Ornstein (1864) informed the Berlin Anthropologic Society that a man of colossal build nursed his son from one of his strongly developed breasts. The Talmud records the case of a man who, when his wife died leaving him a young infant, could not afford a wet nurse. Then—*mirabile dictu*—his breasts expanded like the breasts of a woman and he suckled his son. (Greenblatt, 1972, p.25)

While any of these may be taken with several grains of salt, the article later references far more recent observations of World War II prisoners of war who had been recovering from periods of starvation.

Hibbs, while a captive of the Japanese, personally observed about 500 men with gynecomastia among some 5,000 prisoners; he made note of the fact that galactorrhea was present in a few cases. Jacobs performed a meticulous study of 300 cases of gynecomastia in former war prisoners; there were 9 cases of colostrum-like discharge and one with actual milky secretions. (Greenblatt, 1972, p.33)

Another often cited resource is a chapter of Jared Diamond's *Why is Sex Fun?* where he seems ultimately in favor of or at least neutral on the subject. Although the word *cis* is not used, it is implied by his writing style.

The potential advantages of male lactation are numerous. It would promote a type of emotional bonding of father to child now available only to women. Many men, in fact, are jealous of the special bond arising from breast-feeding, whose traditional restriction to mothers makes men feel excluded. (Diamond, 1997, p.61)

As far as I can see, no formal studies for the purpose of trying to get cis men to lactate have been done, but, in theory, there is no reason why any healthy, adult cis man should not be able to induce lactation if he chooses. Furthermore, the medications and conditions that can cause spontaneous lactation, which I describe in Chapter 10, do not usually have to do with a person's sex or gender and could therefore affect anyone. However, many men who have these conditions may never experience galactorrhea if they don't regularly experience extensive nipple stimulation. So to the first question, "Can any cis man lactate?", I would give the answer of a qualified "yes," for the most part, although medical or mechanical interventions will often be required.

As to the question of why they would want to, it seems reasonable to believe that cis men want to lactate for the same reasons as anyone else. Which is to say, usually to feed and bond with their baby and to a lesser extent for curiosity, fun, or sexual gratification.

For cis men who wish to induce lactation, it's safe to assume the process would be largely the same as for anyone else, only more intense. Consistent pumping on a very strict schedule (at least eight times a day with no longer than a six-hour gap at night), keeping hydrated and getting your vitamins so your body knows it has nutrients to spare, and probably taking hormone treatments or other medications or supplements. This would be for several more months than AFAB people and women who have already been taking hormone treatments. It is impossible to say how many men have done this, given that people would often have to be discreet. However, this excerpt from a letter written to Laura Shanley, included in her essay "Milkmen: Fathers who breastfeed," about two men preparing for their surrogate child, shows that at least a few are doing this, although they find secrecy prudent. Bear in mind that this is a third-person account, but I expect it is mostly true, if somewhat exaggerated.

> The guys were adamant that the baby should get breastmilk. So when she was in her 7th month we bought a really good quality breastpump and Ian started pumping, every 2 hours during the day and once during the night. He was wonderful about it! He used an SNS (supplemental nursing system) after she was born, with donated milk from several friends who were nursing. He was making milk but not a full supply. By the time the baby was 12 weeks old he was

making a full milk supply! He stayed at home with the baby (he was a massage therapist) and nursed her exclusively until she was 8 months old!! I don't think many people outside their intimate circle knew about it, I'm sure folks would have had a fit if they'd known... but I thought it was wonderful! (Shanley, 2017)

Not much has been written on cis men lactating for curiosity or erotic purposes; however, I would not be surprised if this is because anyone interested in it would quickly learn just how much work it involves. I know there are quite a few cis men out there who use electric pumps whether or not any milk comes out, and this seems to scratch their proverbial itch.

In 2011, *Slate* published an article by Michael Thomsen documenting his attempt to lactate just to see if he could. His experience, I expect, is a good example of most cis men who have the same thought.

As the days went on, the comfort turned into monotony. The happy surprise of those first few upward pulls became predictable, a mechanical intrusion into my workday. I couldn't afford the electric pumps, which can cost up to $300, and had to settle for a manual one. It was impossible to do anything useful while holding the pump's suction cup to my chest with one hand and operating the handle with the other. I struggled with the routine, and the loss of at least two or three productive hours each day. (Thomsen, 2011)

He definitely attempted it in the least convenient way possible, and I can't help but wonder how it would have worked out if he had bought a double-sided electric pump.

While I do not expect there will be a great influx of cis men seeking the help of lactation consultants any time soon, we know from these pieces that there is some interest both among researchers and certain of us. Whatever the cause; whether intentionally inducing, or as a spontaneous condition, there seems to be no downside to cis men lactating, and, when you look at the human species as a whole, the practice seems only to be beneficial. I hope this essay will clear up some common misconceptions about who can produce milk, and what kind of men try to find out.

A Queer Person's Guide to Becoming a Lactation Consultant

One of the most important things that we need to talk about when we talk about becoming a lactation consultant (LC) is *what do we mean when we say LC*? In many places, any human being can start advertising services as an LC and it is both technically and legally correct. There's a lot of debate and nuance to the question of whether LCs should be required to be licensed; I find it surprising that so many professions do, but the people in charge of making sure newborns are getting enough to eat do not.

So what is the distinction of being an LC if anyone can do it? There are a few organizations that offer lactation training (usually offering a certification of lactation educator, counselor or coach) but there is no standardization in the curriculum. This is basically the entire point of International Board Certified Lactation Consultants (IBCLC), which is a certification that was developed by some Le Leche League leaders back in 1985. People refer to IBCLC being the gold-standard for lactation support, which is pretty much true since, as of right now, degree programs in human lactation are few and far between.

For many people, the initial interest in becoming a lactation consultant is piqued the first time they meet one, which is usually at the time when they need one most. Bryna discuss this experience in their own life:

> I got pregnant unexpectedly, I didn't know that my migraine med-ication interacted with my birth control [*the medication is called* topiramate, *it is also prescribed for epilepsy and weight* loss]. I decided to go forward with the pregnancy after a lot of agonizing. I had hyperemesis gravidarum so, it was a lot of agonizing in lots of ways. And that experience was dysphoric in a lot of ways, but I didn't really have the words or language specific to my experience at that time. And my ex-partner was not like a terribly amazing person, although that's a different story for a different time. But I ended up really forging a lot of community connections on my own through that pregnancy, through birth and through lactation. And I found a couple of amazing pieces of community, specifically with my lac-tation consultant who started my strong interest in lactation when I was chestfeeding and said, "You'd be amazing at this," and brought me to some educational conferences and took me under her wing as a mentor.

For those of you who are thinking about getting into professional lactation support but currently work in a totally different field, wel-come. I was a professional wine and cheese guy before I decided to pursue my dream of infant care. The following is an excerpt from a piece I was asked to write for the journal, *Clinical Lactation*, "How and why I became an IBCLC."

> Even in my grubby punk rock days I would volunteer to babysit when my friends needed someone and spend the day hanging out downtown with a baby on my hip. So when I was deciding what I wanted to do with my life, I figured out what my ideal job would be and then learned the term for it: postpartum doula. I had actu-ally looked into being a doula some time before but the people I

emailed informed me that only women can be doulas. Not wanting to step on anyone's toes, I took the hint and wrote it off. Apparently, things had changed in the 10 or 15 years since. In 2016, we were living in a major city, so a postpartum doula training was not hard to come by and they were excited to have a man want to attend. The training was disappointing, they spoke a lot about non-judgmental support but followed up with ways for assessing your client's personality traits in order to get them to do what you want. However, it did introduce me to a whole community I did not know existed. I later met the owner of a small doula agency who had a baby on the way herself. She asked me to be her birth doula so I found a birth doula training and attended my first and only birth. I realized that as excited as the community was to have a guy taking a serious interest in birthwork and infant care, I could not make a living as either kind of doula without expanding. I attended a seminar called something like, "Who wants to be an IBCLC?" where I received an overview of the certification process which, as we know, can be daunting for an outsider. The organizer later offered me a position as a secretary with the understanding that I would be able to learn about different aspects of infant care and have the opportunity to meet parents who might need help at home. I did not realize at the time how lucky a break that was. When my supervisor encouraged me to start formal IBCLC training (Pathway 3) I had all the clinical hours I would need, not realizing that for many people finding a clinical mentor is the most difficult part of the training.

The training itself went about as well as could be expected. Not having a medical background, I was pleased to learn that most of the credits I needed were available online as well as the lactation education. The lactation and birthworker community was overall supportive, I low-grade expected to be yelled at a few times, but the worst I experienced was occasional condescension, which has waned since I've become more of a known entity. Over the few years it took me to complete my training and take the International

Board of Lactation Consultant Examiners exam (I was in the cohort whose tests were postponed due to the Covid-19 pandemic), I started teaching childbirth classes for first-time fathers. I realized how much I loved teaching people about this kind of thing. I also started learning about the intersection of the queer aspects of my life and lactation support. As I learned about induced lactation, I also learned that LGBTQIA+ and polyamorous families often have no idea this is something they can do. As I learned about chest surgeries, I realized that trans masculine people are not given information about how top surgery will affect their ability to lactate should they decide to give birth later. I learned all of these amazing things that the people who could benefit most from have no idea exist. (Engelsman, 2023)

As I described in my article above, getting an IBCLC qualification has four main components: lactation education, bona fide college credits, supervised clinical hours, and a test.

- *95 hours of lactation education.* The International Board of Lactation Consultant Examiners (IBLCE), which is the governing body behind the IBCLC, is pretty lax when it comes to this education. They don't have a detailed list of approved organizations, although a lot of the companies that offer LC training will say that people have used their course for IBCLC certification. A great many people will take one of these courses, then begin offering services as a lactation coach or counselor. This is fine as long as they don't call themselves an IBCLC. There is no standard for the curriculum taught in these courses, so you will definitely want to vet any courses you are interested in to make sure they meet *your* standards.

- *14 college credits.* These are all 101 or 102 level courses: biology, statistics, anatomy, sociology, that sort of thing. There are several websites where you can take the courses, and, as long as they will grant you transferable credits, you should be fine.

- *300–1000 clinical hours.* The number of hours you need depends on your experience—the organization refers to this as pathways.

    - Pathway 1 is for those who are already medical professionals. You will need 1000 hours but they don't need to be supervised.

    - Pathway 2 can be done at some colleges which offer lactation certificate programs where you can get all of the education and hours over the course of a few years. This streamlines the process, but is generally a more expensive option.

    - Pathway 3 is if you're doing everything piecemeal. You need 500 hours but you also need a mentor to supervise you. This is the really hard part for most prospective IBCLCs, especially if you also need to have a job. A lot of IBCLCs don't pay their interns, and some will even expect you to pay them! And, of course, you never know if available mentors are going to be supportive of queer clients or interns. If you live in an area without many options, you may want to look into broadening your search since clinical hours can also be acquired from online consultations.

- *The test.* The test is given two times per year and is different every time. However, there are always 175 multiple choice questions, more than half of which involve identifying photos of infant behavior or various medical conditions. What constitutes a passing grade changes every time and different questions are weighted differently, so it takes a long time to find out if you have passed or not. You used to have to retake the test every ten years, but they recently changed the rules so you can recertify by getting 75 CERPs (continuing education credits) every five years instead.

As I mentioned, Le Leche League (LLL) is the founding body of the IBLCE, as well as a common route for applicants to get their clinical hours. Unfortunately, the organization does not have a great history with gender-inclusive support; however, changes have been made in the recent past. Kristin-Cole was instrumental in making those changes happen, as they discussed in our interview:

I was a leader, and I was a queer leader, and I was one of the only queer leaders. There were literally a handful of us and we were doxxed, we were threatened, we were constantly having complaints written against us from the Board of Directors. This was from probably ten, eleven years ago all the way through to this past year when I finally left. I mean, the Board of Directors were making complaints and harassing us—really vile, vile stuff. It's been the single biggest source of anti-queer bias in my life.

We made three huge steps. We got the Father Concept changed, to be more inclusive and to talk about all the different support people for the birthing parent. We got LLL's style manual changed, so that they would alternate uses of the word *mother* and more gender neutral terms. And the thing that finally made me feel that it was okay for me to put it down was, the LLL book; their sort of Bible, called *The Womanly Art of Breastfeeding*. It has been called this since the 1950s. And they finally agreed to rename it with the next edition that's going to come out. It's just gonna be called *The Art of Breastfeeding*. That was ten years of basically 20 people being kind of tortured in a lot of really intense ways. It was really bad. And so, basically, once those three things happened, and they happened pretty quickly in succession, after a lot of work, I felt much more at peace with the decision that I felt like it was time and that I had accomplished as much as I could possibly accomplish. I felt at peace with the decision, finally. I'd spent a lot of years being like, well, they're gonna have to kick me out. And they almost did several times because I wouldn't stop criticizing them. But we accomplished the things that we worked hard to accomplish and so I felt good about that. But yeah, it was really, really hard. And trust me, I was not alone in it. There was a core group that worked our asses off and made a lot of sacrifices.

The Father Concept that they refer to was one of the original ten concepts LLL was founded on. The original text read: "The father's role in the breastfeeding relationship is one of provider, protector, helpmate and companion to the mother; by thus supporting her he enables her to mother the baby more completely." The updated text reads, "Breastfeeding is enhanced by the loving support of the baby's father, a co-parent, a partner, and/or close family members who value the breastfeeding relationship" (Guzmán, 2021).

References

APILAM (Association for Promotion of and Cultural and Scientific Research into Breastfeeding). (2002). e-lactancia. Accessed on 08/08/2023 at https://e-lactancia.org

Armstrong, M.L., Caliendo, C., & Roberts, AE. (2006). Pregnancy, lactation and nipple piercings. *AWHONN Lifelines, 10*(3), 212–217. https://doi.org/10.1111/j.1552-6356.2006.00034.x

Aronson, J.K. (2016). Psilocybin. *Meyler's Side Effects of Drugs*. 1048–1051. https://doi.org/10.1016/b978-0-444-53717-1.00158-x

Berens, P., Eglash, A., Malloy, M., & Steube, A.M. (2016). ABM Clinical Protocol #26: Persistent Pain with Breastfeeding. *Breastfeeding Medicine, 11*(2), 46–53. https://doi.org/10.1089/bfm.2016.29002.pjb

Berens, P. & Labbok, M. (2015). ABM Clinical Protocol #13: Contraception During Breastfeeding, Revised 2015. *Breastfeeding Medicine, 10*(1), 3–12. https://doi.org/10.1089/bfm.2015.9999

Brodribb, W. (2018). ABM Clinical Protocol #9: Use of Galactogogues in Initiating or Augmenting Maternal Milk Production, Second Revision 2018. *Breastfeeding Medicine, 13*(5), 307–314. https://doi.org/10.1089/bfm.2018.29092.wjb

Cheng, F., Dai, S., Wang, C., Zeng, S., Chen, J., & Cen, Y. (2018). Do breast implants influence breastfeeding? A meta-analysis of comparative studies. *Journal of Human Lactation, 34*(3), 424–432. https://doi.org/10.1177/0890334418776654

Deakin University. (2019). *Breastfeeding hormones in play* [Video]. YouTube. www.youtube.com/watch?v=6ECZnmcgHOc

Diamond, J.M. (1997). *Why is Sex Fun?: The Evolution of Human Sexuality*. Basic Books.

Eliot, L. (2010). *What's Going on in There?* Bantam.

Engelsman, J. (2023). Commentary: How and why I became an IBCLC. *Clinical Lactation, 14*(2), 43–44. https://doi.org/10.1891/cl-2023-0004

Erickson-Schroth, L. (2022). *Trans Bodies, Trans Selves: A Resource by and for Transgender Communities*. Oxford University Press.

Facelli, V. (2023). *Feed the Baby: An Inclusive Guide to Nursing, Bottle-Feeding, and Everything in Between*. The Countryman Press.

Feinstein, B.A. & Dyar, C. (2017). Bisexuality, minority stress, and health. *Current Sexual Health Reports, 9*(1), 42–49. https://doi.org/10.1007/s11930-017-0096-3

Garbin, C.P., Deacon, J.P., Rowan, M.K., Hartmann, P.E., & Geddes, D.T. (2009). Association of nipple piercing with abnormal milk production and breastfeeding. *JAMA, 301*(24), 2550. https://doi.org/10.1001/jama.2009.877

Glick, J.L., Andrinopoulos, K.M., Theall, K.P., & Kendall, C. (2018). "Tiptoeing around the system": Alternative healthcare navigation among gender minorities in New Orleans. *Transgender Health, 3*(1), 118–126. https://doi.org/10.1089/trgh.2018.0015

Goldfarb, L. & Newman, J. (2002). *The Newman-Goldfarb Protocols for Induced Lactation*. Ask Lenor. Accessed on 08/28/2024 at https://www.asklenore.info/breastfeeding/induced-lactation

Greenblatt, R. (1972). Inappropriate lactation in men and women. *Medical Aspects of Human Sexuality, 6*(6), 25–33.

Guzmán, H. (2021, July 2). The Evolution of the Support Concept. *Le Leche League International*. Accessed on 08/31/2023 at https://llli.org/news/the-evolution-of-the-support-concept

Hunt, M.J., Salisbury, E., Grace, J., & Armati, R.P. (1996). Black breast milk due to minocycline therapy. *British Journal of Dermatology, 134*(5), 943–944. https://doi.org/10.1046/j.1365-2133.1996.134869.x

Jewell, M.L., Edwards, M.C., Murphy, D.K., & Schumacher, A. (2019). Lactation outcomes in more than 3500 women following primary augmentation: 5-year data from the Breast Implant Follow-Up Study. *Aesthetic Surgery Journal, 39*(8), 875–883. https://doi.org/10.1093/asj/sjy221

Johnson, H.M., Eglash, A., Mitchell, K.B., Leeper, K., *et al.* (2020). ABM Clinical Protocol #32: Management of Hyperlactation. *Breastfeeding Medicine, 15*(3), 129–134. https://doi.org/10.1089/bfm.2019.29141.hmj

Jones, E. & Warner, H. (2023). *Antenatal hand expression*. Buckinghamshire Healthcare NHS Trust, Birth Choices Website. Accessed on 08/31/2023 at www.buckshealthcare.nhs.uk/birthchoices/pifs/antenatal-hand-expression

Kali, K.L. (2022). *Queer Conception*. Sasquatch Books.

Kamali, A., Jamieson, D.J., Kpaduwa, J., Schrier, S., *et al.* (2016). Pregnancy, labor, and delivery after ebola virus disease and implications for infection control in obstetric services, United States. *Emerging Infectious Diseases, 22*(7). https://doi.org/10.3201/eid2207.160269

Laozi. (2008). *Tao Te Ching*. Shambhala.

LeFort, Y., Evans, A., Livingstone, V., Douglas, P., *et al.* (2021). Academy of

Breastfeeding Medicine Position Statement on Ankyloglossia in Breastfeeding Dyads. *Breastfeeding Medicine, 16*(4), 278–281. https://doi.org/10.1089/bfm.2021.29179.ylf

Li, R., Dee, D., Li, C.-M., Hoffman, H.J., & Grummer-Strawn, L.M. (2014). Breastfeeding and risk of infections at 6 years. *Pediatrics, 134*(Supplement), S13–S20. https://doi.org/10.1542/peds.2014-0646d

Meek, J.Y. & Noble, L. (2022). Policy Statement: Breastfeeding and the Use of Human Milk. *Pediatrics, 150*(1). https://doi.org/10.1542/peds.2022-057988

Mitchell, K.B., Johnson, H.M., Eglash, A., Young, M., *et al.* (2019). ABM Clinical Protocol #30: Breast Masses, Breast Complaints, and Diagnostic Breast Imaging in the Lactating Woman. *Breastfeeding Medicine, 14*(4), 208–214. https://doi.org/10.1089/bfm.2019.29124.kjm

Mortel, M. & Mehta, S.D. (2013). Systematic review of the efficacy of herbal galactogogues. *Journal of Human Lactation, 29*(2), 154–162. https://doi.org/10.1177/0890334413477243

Moyo, G.T., Thomas-Jackson, S.C., Childress, A., Dawson, J., *et al.* (2021). Chrononutrition and breast milk: A review of the circadian variation of hormones present in human milk. *Clinical Lactation, 12*(3), 114–123. https://doi.org/10.1891/clinlact-d-20-00035

Murkoff, H. (2024). *What to Expect When You're Expecting* (6th edition). Simon and Schuster.

National Health Service. (2020, December 7). *Your breastfeeding questions answered*. NHS.UK. Accessed on 08/31/2023 at www.nhs.uk/conditions/baby/breastfeeding-and-bottle-feeding/breastfeeding/your-questions-answered

National Health Service. (2023, March 21). *HIV and Feeding Your Baby*. University Hospitals Sussex NHS Foundation Trust. Accessed on 08/09/2023 at www.uhsussex.nhs.uk/resources/hiv-and-feeding-your-baby

Oberhelman-Eaton, S., Chang, A., Gonzalez, C., Braith, A., *et al.* (2021). Initiation of gender-affirming testosterone therapy in a lactating transgender man. *Journal of Human Lactation, 38*(2), 339–343. https://doi.org/10.1177/08903344211037646

Panel on Treatment of HIV During Pregnancy and Prevention of Perinatal Transmission. (2023). *Recommendations for the Use of Antiretroviral Drugs During Pregnancy and Interventions to Reduce Perinatal HIV Transmission in the United States.* Department of Health and Human Services. Accessed on 08/09/2023 at https://clinicalinfo.hiv.gov/en/guidelines/perinatal

Reece-Stremtan, S., Campos, M., Kokajko, L., Brodribb, W., *et al.* (2017). ABM Clinical Protocol #15: Analgesia and Anesthesia for the Breastfeeding Mother, Revised 2017. *Breastfeeding Medicine, 12*(9), 500–506. https://doi.org/10.1089/bfm.2017.29054.srt

Reece-Stremtan, S. & Marinelli, K.A. (2015). ABM Clinical Protocol #21: Guidelines for Breastfeeding and Substance Use or Substance Use Disorder,

Revised 2015. *Breastfeeding Medicine, 10*(3), 135–141. https://doi.org/10.1089/bfm.2015.9992

Ruddle, L. (2020). *Relactation: A Guide to Rebuilding Your Milk Supply.* Praeclarus Press.

Schnell, A. (2013). *Breastfeeding Without Birthing: A Breastfeeding Guide for Mothers Through Adoption, Surrogacy, and Other Special Circumstances.* Praeclarus Press.

Schnell, A. (2022). The three step framework for inducing lactation™. *Journal of Human Lactation, 38*(2), 252–261. https://doi.org/10.1177/08903344221076531

Shanley, L. (2017). *Milkmen: Fathers who breastfeed.* In *Unassisted Childbirth.* 3rd ed. Accessed on 09/05/2023 at https://unassistedchildbirth.com/inspiration/milkmen-fathers-who-breastfeed

Silver, AJ. (2022). *Supporting Queer Birth.* London: Jessica Kingsley Publishers.

Silver, AJ. (2024). *Supporting Fat Birth.* London: Jessica Kingsley Publishers.

Skovlund, C.W., Mørch, L.S., Kessing, L.V., & Lidegaard, Ø. (2016). Association of hormonal contraception with Depression. *JAMA Psychiatry, 73*(11), 1154–1162. https://doi.org/10.1001/jamapsychiatry.2016.2387

Sriraman, N.K., Melvin, K., & Meltzer-Brody, S. (2015). ABM Clinical Protocol #18: Use of Antidepressants in Breastfeeding Mothers. *Breastfeeding Medicine, 10*(6), 290–299. https://doi.org/10.1089/bfm.2015.29002

Thompson, R.F. (1990). *Requiem for the Degas of the B-Boys, Keith Haring.* Artforum. Accessed on 09/12/2023, at www.artforum.com/print/199005/requiem-for-the-degas-of-the-b-boys-keith-haring-34080

Thomsen, M. (2011). Man milk: My curious quest to breast-feed. *Slate.* Accessed on 09/05/2023 at https://slate.com/technology/2011/05/male-lactation-can-a-33-year-old-guy-learn-to-breast-feed.html

Wambach, K. & Spencer, B. (2019). *Breastfeeding and Human Lactation.* Jones & Bartlett Learning.

Weaver, L.W. (2021). *White Blood: A History of Human Milk: How Babies have been Fed from Antiquity to Modern Times and Why it Matters.* Unicorn.

West, D. (2008). *Clinics in Human Lactation: Breastfeeding After Breast and Nipple Procedures: A Guide for Healthcare Professionals.* Hale Publishing.

Whisenhunt, D. & Atlanta New First Staff. (2024, January 27). Fire at Decatur gender clinic was intentional, being investigated as hate crime. Accessed on 02/15/2024 at www.atlantanewsfirst.com/2024/01/27/fire-decatur-gender-clinic-was-intentional-being-investigated-as-hate-crime.

Wiessinger, D., West, D., Smith, L.J., & Pitman, T. (2014). *Sweet Sleep.* Ballantine Books.

Wilson-Clay, B. & Hoover, K. (2017). *The Breastfeeding Atlas.* Lactnews Press.

Witkowska-Zimny, M., Kamińska-El-Hassan, E., & Wróbel, E. (2019). Milk therapy: Unexpected uses for human breast milk. *Nutrients, 11*(5), 944. https://doi.org/10.3390/nu11050944

World Health Organization. (1998). The World Health Organization multinational study of breast-feeding and lactational amenorrhea. I. Description of infant feeding patterns and of the return of menses. *Fertility and Sterility, 70*(3), 448–460. https://doi.org/10.1016/s0015-0282(98)00190-3

World Health Organization & United Nations Children's Fund. (2016). *Guideline: Updates on HIV and Infant Feeding: The duration of breastfeeding and support from health services to improve feeding practices among mothers living with HIV.* World Health Organization. Accessed on 08/09/2023 at https://apps.who.int/iris/bitstream/handle/10665/246260/9789241549707-eng.pdf

World Health Organization. (2021). *Breastfeeding.* World Health Organization. Accessed on 08/31/2023 at www.who.int/health-topics/breastfeeding#tab=tab_2

Wright, R. (2019). *Baby-Friendly USA: About Us.* Baby-Friendly USA. Accessed on 08/09/2023 at www.babyfriendlyusa.org/about

Notes

Supporting Fat Birth

A Book for Birth Professionals and Parents

AJ Silver

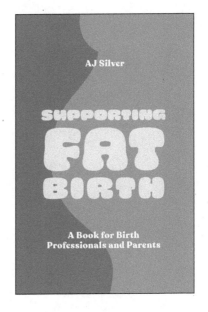

This pioneering guide provides birth professionals, pregnant people, and advocates with comprehensive insight into navigating conception, pregnancy, birth, and the perinatal period whilst fat. Drawing on the author's decade of experience as well as evidence-based research and case studies from people sharing their own perspectives and stories, this authoritative and compassionate book provides practical and effective advice on how to improve quality of care for fat parents. It covers a wide range of topics across the birth journey and beyond including interviews with a number of high-profile people including Nicola Salmon and Amber Marshall and empowers readers to feel reassured and confident in their choices and rights. This ground-breaking resource challenges the pervasive bias against fat service users in the birthing world and acts as a call to action to dismantle the fatphobic stigma present in our healthcare systems in order to create an environment that is inclusive of all bodies.

£26.99 | $35 | PB | 224PP | ISBN 978 1 83997 633 9 | eISBN 978 1 83997 634 6

A Doula's Guide to Improving Maternal Health for BIPOC Women

Jacquelyn Clemmons

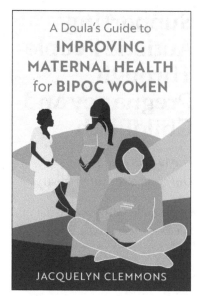

Women of color are at far more risk of serious complications during pregnancy and childbirth through factors relating to racism, sexism, income inequality, and a lack of access to resources. This invaluable guide equips birth workers with the training and knowledge to provide holistic, person-centered care for their clients of all backgrounds.

You'll learn how to serve the specific needs of your clients, how to advocate for them as they navigate the challenges many black and brown women face, and how to understand your client's pain points whilst also nourishing yourself and maintaining a good business structure. Your emotional and spiritual wellbeing as a birth worker is of vital importance and this guide will nourish you in your training just as you learn how to support and advocate for others. It will provide several options on business structures so you may cater to clients from all backgrounds and also includes pre- and post-birth grounding techniques for you, your clients, and their families.

£19.99 | $27.95 | PB | 160PP | ISBN 978 1 83997 176 1 | eISBN 978 1 83997 177 8

Supporting Autistic People Through Pregnancy and Childbirth

Hayley Morgan, Emma Durman, and Karen Henry

Forewords by Carly Jones, Wenn B. Lawson, and Sheena Byrom

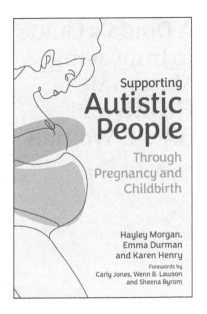

This comprehensive and accessible guide is for every birthing and health professional looking to improve their care during pregnancy, birth, and aftercare for autistic women. With a distinct lack of scientifically approached work in this area, this much-needed book takes an intersectional, feminist approach and covers the background of modern birth practices and autism as a diagnosis.

With intersectionality as a core feature, the impact of cultural differences, underdiagnoses, stigma, and stereotypes amongst ethnic minorities is also included. It discusses how pain functions in the autistic brain as well as co-occurring conditions such as alexithymia, chronic pain, epilepsy, and Ehlers-Danlos Syndrome. This multidisciplinary author team includes two well-established autism experts, and an experienced midwife and lecturer who provides invaluable birthing insight, as well as approaches for sensation management during birth, insider knowledge on midwifery protocols, and accessible tools for autistic pregnant people and families to use.

£26.99 | $35 | PB | 304PP | ISBN 978 1 83997 105 1 | eISBN 978 1 83997 106 8